QUICK AND EASY

LOW-FAT RECIPES

FROM AROUND THE WORLD

ANNOUK VAN DE VOORDE

≡People's Medical Society®

Allentown, Pennsylvania

The People's Medical Society is a nonprofit consumer health organization dedicated to the principles of better, more responsive and less expensive medical care. Organized in 1983, the People's Medical Society puts previously unavailable medical information into the hands of consumers so that they can make informed decisions about their own health care.

Membership in the People's Medical Society is $20 a year and includes a subscription to the *People's Medical Society Newsletter.* For information, write to the People's Medical Society, 462 Walnut Street, Allentown, PA 18102, or call 610-770-1670.

This and other People's Medical Society publications are available for quantity purchase at discount. Contact the People's Medical Society for details.

Many of the designations used by manufacturers and sellers to distinguish their products are claimed as trademarks. Where those designations appear in this book and the People's Medical Society was aware of a trademark claim, the designations have been printed in initial capital letters (e.g., Jell-O).

© 1997 by the People's Medical Society
Printed in the United States of America

Cover photograph © George G. Weiser, 1996
Design by Jerry O'Brien
Nutritional analyses provided by Winter Springs Editorial Services

Library of Congress Cataloging-in-Publication Data

Van de Voorde, Annouk.
    Quick and easy low-fat recipes from around the world / Annouk Van de Voorde.
        p. cm.
    Includes index.
    ISBN 1-882606-65-5
    1. Cookery, International. 2. Low-fat diet—Recipes. 3. Low-calorie diet—Recipes. 4. Quick and easy cookery. I. Title.
TX725.A1M33   1997
641.5'638—dc20   96-36055
                                                                CIP

1 2 3 4 5 6 7 8 9 0
First printing, January 1997

To my son, Thierry, and my daughter, Tatiana, for being so health-conscious and for choosing professions dedicated to health

CONTENTS

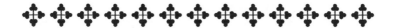

INTRODUCTION

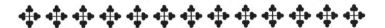

When I was growing up, I was strictly forbidden to use four-letter words.

And *diet* was one of them!

The word is obsolete. It conjured images of quarantine or incarceration for breaking the law. It set me apart as though I had the plague.

Alas, I was born and raised with fat cells. So was my entire family.

We, the children of pioneering parents, were raised on a quinine and coffee plantation in Rwanda, surrounded by exotic, sun-ripened fruits and vegetables. My mother had trained our *pichi* (Swahili for "cook") to cook the Belgian way: mouthwatering, butter-drenched crème fraîche and wine-based, rich sauces—not to mention her baba au rhum! Five or six courses at a sitting. We entertained a lot.

Because we lived deep in equatorial Africa during those crucial pioneering days, my parents doubled their efforts in "force-feeding" us just in case we'd succumb to dysentery or malaria or bilharziasis. I do believe we survived those tender years only because we had extra padding. My father, who had served in the French Foreign Legion, told us about Middle Eastern cuisine. Our Portuguese neighbor taught us how to stew a good calderata with potatoes, codfish, tomatoes, onions, liters of olive oil and so much garlic we had to sequester the whole family.

After the revolution I went to live in Europe. Ah, the Belgian waffles dripping with butter, glazed with gooey brown sugar! And that wicked Lady Godiva inducing men and even women into sin!

Later, when I was to live in Johannesburg, South Africa, I learned not only to speak English but also to eat steak and kidney pie, skewered lamb with crackling skin, boer wurst bursting with grease.

The tides of my life brought me to America, where I dealt with juicy hamburgers and hot dogs and mounds of pastrami veined with solid fat. I discovered olive-studded bologna. How good life was, so replete. So *fat*.

My way of coping was to go on fasting binges until my head spun and I had to sit on a street curb because I was so faint. At least I was not on a diet. I was simply starving. Youth is forgiving.

Later I married a Greek man, who taught me the wonders of Greek cooking. I spent endless hours in the kitchen baking spanakopita, baklava and rich, oh-so-rich kourabiedes filled with nuts and butter. I still salivate at the memory.

Let it be known that one sin I did not commit was to pass on fat cells to my children. Soon after their births, I joined a weight-reduction group and learned a *new way of life*. This led to a new career. I became a class lecturer and moderator. The highlight of my classes was to distribute recipes from around the world created especially for my students using the techniques of the weight-reducing group.

My motto has always been: *no deprivation*. Why subject myself to limp vegetables or a truckload of crunchy vegetables? I am not a rabbit. I am a slim, size-8 woman in her fifties who demands elegant food. Who entertains with low-fat, international foods. I must have my curries, my soufflés, my coq au vin. I indulge in one glass of dry wine a day, but it must be served in a crystal goblet. When I eat, I chew slowly, and I listen to Vivaldi. Or Chopin. I will always be obsessed with food, but I have directed that missile into creative thinking patterns about food.

My sweet punishment when I occasionally go astray is to walk an extra mile. Or to jump rope for 10 minutes. Or to do my stairs 10 times, up and down. There are millions of ways to shed pounds but only one way to get fat.

Now that I live in Mexico, I am gorging myself on freshly made tortillas! And black beans and jicama with the most piquant of sauces. Every day is a food fiesta. To counterbalance my *dolce vita*, I do weights at the local gym. I am the only woman in her fifties to do it here.

My grown children, Thierry and Tatiana, are both engaged in health-related professions. They work out, jog, row, ski, water-ski. My son even dared skydiving, jumping off the top of one of Rio de Janeiro's peaks. Indeed, they are chips off their mother's block: They have learned to eat well—low-fat, low-salt but superbly elegant international foods. It is easy to "decalorize" just about every recipe.

We cannot deny our culture. Eating is about the most "cultural" pastime and one of the only excitements that never wanes. International food makes you go places without ever leaving your doorstep. It is the fuel that keeps your body running.

We want to live a thousand lives to do all of the things we'd like to do. But we want to have our cake and eat it, too! We want to remain healthy, energetic and slim while continuing to adore food.

INGREDIENTS IN THE CUPBOARD

I consider food ingredients like a wardrobe. You can rely on some basic ingredients because their tastes are classic and can be depended upon. For the more exotic dishes, I expand my basics to include a variety of fresh herbs in season and dried ingredients in winter. Or whatever's appropriate to a particular country's custom.

A good nonstick skillet is the most valuable tool for low-fat, low-calorie cooking. I urge you to make that investment. A blender and/or a food processor is also a basic necessity. A blender converts any leftovers in the fridge into a succulent soup or dip. It makes bread crumbs and a horde of other fast dishes. It is simply magical!

Arrowroot and cornstarch: I use these in moderation to make sauces. One tablespoon of either will thicken 1 cup of skim milk for a white sauce. I have given instructions on how to do this in the appropriate recipes.

Bacon bits: For those of us who cannot do without that bacon taste. They come in jars and shakers and can be found at spice counters.

Bread crumbs: Toast or bake the bread. Let it dry a bit. Break it into a blender container and blend to the desired consistency.

Breads: All of the latest research indicates that only whole-grain breads should be used. There are so many tasty choices today.

Cheeses: Lately there has been a great improvement in the taste and availability of low-fat cheeses. You can find a low-fat version of virtually any type of cheese.

Chicken seasoning: Many of my recipes call for this basic ingredient. There are three varieties that are interchangeable in flavor and calorie counts.

• Chicken-flavored instant broth and seasoning: a yellow powder sold in envelopes (one envelope can be used for each teaspoon of chicken seasoning).

• Chicken-flavored instant bouillon: a brown granular powder in jars, found where bouillon cubes are sold. Use as instructed.

• Chicken stock base: a light yellow powder sold in jars.

Chives: Always use fresh chives when available. The freeze-dried kind sold in bottles at spice counters can be substituted, but in half of the portion. If these are not available, you can use a green onion, minced.

Cooking-oil sprays: I use these only when necessary and recommend the olive oil or canola oil varieties. Just a fine spray at the bottom of the pan will prevent the food from adhering to it.

Garlic: I use a lot of garlic. It runs in my blood, and the latest research seems to indicate that it makes your blood run. I always use the minced fresh variety. When I call for garlic powder, it is for reasons of consistency in a particular dish. Garlic powder is not garlic salt! They cannot be substituted for each other. Remember that one key to health is low salt!

Milk: For all recipes that call for skim milk, I prefer to use evaporated skim milk because it imparts a creamy taste. It is interchangeable with skim milk. When a recipe calls for dry milk, it means powdered skim milk to which no water is added. Lately I have used soy milk in some of my preparations. When it's blended with other condiments, I cannot taste the difference.

Oils and fats: The secret to low-fat cooking is to add the oil/butter/fat just before serving. A teaspoon goes a long way, and because it is topical, it hits the palate before anything else. Use olive oil (the first-pressed oil) whenever possible.

Rice: Often my recipes call for 1/2 cup of white rice. To prepare 1/2 cup successfully, use this method:

> In a small nonstick saucepan put 1/2 cup of water, 1/8 teaspoon of salt and 3 level tablespoons of regular long-grain white rice. Bring to a boil without stirring. Cover and immediately reduce the heat to the lowest setting. Cook for 15 minutes. This yields 1/2 cup— and a mere 100 calories.

Salt: This book recommends low-salt products. For most of us a small amount of salt is healthy. For those of you who cannot use salt at all, please ask for your doctor's recommendation. There are some excellent salt substitute products on the market, but use these only with medical counsel. Also, try to use more pepper and lemon, herbs and salt-free condiments.

Sesame oil: You can buy it at an Asian grocery or a health food store. Or try the Asian food counter at the supermarket. Like olive oil, a few drops will impart a succulent, rich taste. The best color is dark brown.

Sugars: I use only honey, raw sugar, fructose or the new "jam" or "marmalade" variety, sweetened with fruit juice. Your choice. If your doctor recommends a sugar substitute, remember to use just enough to impart that sweet taste!

Tomato sauce: Only the canned variety, without oil or sweeteners. Tomato puree is also good and may be substituted. I don't use tomato paste in my recipes because it imparts a different, concentrated flavor.

White cheeses: Low-fat cottage cheese, low-fat ricotta cheese and low-fat farmer cheese are interchangeable. I much prefer the texture of ricotta cheese. Mozzarella cheese also comes in a low-fat version.

WHAT YOU NEED TO KNOW ABOUT FAT

Before you race to the kitchen, there are a few things you need to know about fats. Read on.

Research has indicated that eating fatty foods contributes to health problems such as high blood pressure, heart disease, stroke, obesity, diabetes and cancer. Experts tell us that in order to maintain maximum health, we should cut down our fat intake. The American Heart Association, the National Cancer Institute, the National Academy of Sciences and the American Health Foundation all recommend that for anyone over two years of age, no more than 30 percent of our daily calories should come from fat. Some nutritional experts urge that our diets be even lower in fat. This doesn't mean that every food or meal that we eat has to be within these guidelines. A higher-fat meal or food can be balanced with lower-fat meals or foods throughout the day.

Below are descriptions of the major dietary fats.

Saturated fats: These fats are usually of animal origin and are solid at room temperature. These are the fats we should avoid, since they are associated with an increased risk of heart disease and possibly cancer. Saturated fats raise the risk of heart disease by contributing to high cholesterol levels; specifically, they raise blood levels of low-density lipoprotein (LDL), the so-called bad cholesterol.

Unsaturated fats: Unsaturated fats are usually of vegetable origin. They are liquid at room temperature and include monounsaturated and polyunsaturated fats.

• Monounsaturated fats: Unlike polyunsaturated fats, these fats are thought to drop levels of the harmful LDL cholesterol without reducing levels of high-density lipoprotein (HDL)—the so-called good cholesterol—improving the body's ability to transport excess fat to the liver for disposal. These fats can be found in olive, canola and peanut oils.

• Polyunsaturated fats: Found in corn, safflower, sunflower, cottonseed, soybean and walnut oils, these fats were once thought to reduce cholesterol levels. However, researchers now believe that these oils decrease levels of HDL, the cholesterol that helps remove fat from the body, while leaving levels of LDL unchanged.

Trans fatty acids: These fats were once thought to be healthier than saturated fats. However, recent research has determined that trans fatty acids act in ways similar to saturated fats—they raise LDL cholesterol levels. You'll find trans fatty acids in hydrogenated vegetable oils, components of margarine and vegetable shortening.

APPETIZERS
AND BEVERAGES

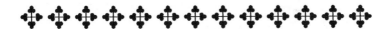

We come home after a hard day's work. This is an important part of the day—and a dangerous one if not tended to. We need comfort and can have it!

What shall it be? How nice to have so many healthy choices today and still be able to lose weight or maintain the weight goal we have already achieved. To go to a table hungry is treading temptation. Also, we want to take a few minutes to prepare the meal. This is the time for an appetizer. Let's indulge: Our bodies and spirits need kindling.

Instead of using bread or crackers for the dips that follow, try carrot sticks, zucchini fingers and fresh cuts of green pepper. If you can find jicama in your neighborhood store (I always did), peel it and cut it into thin slices, raw. It will look like a cracker but crunch and taste like a water chestnut. It is virtually calorie-free and bursting with juice, and it can be spiced to taste. It can be cubed for salads or slivered for a copycat of the French celery *rave* when tossed into a low-fat imitation mayonnaise or your own nonfat vinaigrette. If you add a dash of cumin, you will turn anything into a Middle Eastern feast. Some curry powder will be your odyssey to India. Or a dash of hot cayenne. Or a hot, peppery sauce. The sky is the limit.

If this is the time you want your bread, go ahead! Be sure it is a whole-grain loaf. It gives joy to the palate. We can chew hard and long and lengthen the pleasure and get all of that fiber—not to mention the rich taste and the health benefits.

BALKAN CAVIAR

Nutrition Facts
Number of Servings: 4
Per Serving
- Calories: 112
- Saturated Fat: 0.569 gram
- Monounsaturated Fat: 0.649 gram
- Polyunsaturated Fat: 1.041 grams
- Total Fat: 4.03 grams
- Percentage of Calories From Fat: 34%

Black caviar can be found in every supermarket at a reasonable price. This is a spectacular dish that is bound to get you applause. It's easy and fast to boot!

²/₃ cup low-fat ricotta cheese
1 tbsp. lemon juice
1 tsp. chicken seasoning or your favorite low-salt powdered flavoring
1 tbsp. minced dried onions
4 hard-cooked eggs
2 tsp. fat-free mayonnaise
1 tsp. minced capers, drained (if desired)
3 ½ oz. lumpfish caviar, well drained
Minced fresh parsley or dill for garnish
8 slices whole-grain or whole-wheat bread, toasted and cut into pie-shaped pieces, or 8 tortillas, browned directly over a gas flame or quick toasted (if desired)

1. In a mixing bowl or food processor blend the cheese, lemon juice, chicken seasoning or flavoring and onions until smooth. Chill for 1 hour, or to spread consistency.
2. Discard the yolks from 2 of the eggs and finely grate the remaining 2 yolks and the egg whites. Mix the grated eggs, mayonnaise and capers if using.
3. On an elegant serving platter shape the egg mixture into a patty about 1 inch high. Chill.
4. With a wooden spoon or plastic spatula, spread the caviar over the patty, covering the sides as well. Disguise the caviar with the cheese spread by carefully patting the cheese over the caviar. Garnish with the parsley or dill. This dish will make liquid if made hours in advance. Simply blot up the liquid with paper towels before serving. Serve with the bread or tortillas if using.

A TIP FOR THE COOK

To make your own low-fat mayonnaise, puree ½ cup (4 ounces) of soft tofu, 1 teaspoon of white vinegar, ¼ teaspoon of dry mustard and a pinch of cayenne pepper in a blender jar.

MEXICALI CHILI BEAN DIP

Nutrition Facts
  Number of Servings: 2
  Per Serving
  • Calories: 181
  • Saturated Fat: 0.366 gram
  • Monounsaturated Fat: 0.173 gram
  • Polyunsaturated Fat: 0.48 gram
  • Total Fat: 1.4 grams
  • Percentage of Calories From Fat: 7%

From across the border comes this healthy, fiery dish, which uses three kinds of pepper to season it. Guaranteed to "summerize" those chilly winter nights. The dip can be scooped up with any crunchy vegetable. Olé!

1/3 cup low-fat cottage cheese, ricotta cheese or farmer cheese
1   jar (4 oz.) pimientos, drained (save the liquid)
3   cloves garlic, minced
1/4 cup tomato sauce
1   cup cooked red kidney beans, drained
1   small, hot canned chili pepper (for strong palates only)
    Dash of ground cumin (if available)
1   tsp. chili powder
    Dash of salt (if desired but preferable)
    Lemon juice (if desired but preferable)

1. In a blender jar combine all of the ingredients except the salt and lemon juice, starting with the cheese at the bottom. Blend until smooth. If it's too thick, add some of the pimiento liquid until the desired consistency is reached.
2. Season with the salt and lemon juice if using.

HUMMUS

Nutrition Facts
Number of Servings: 2
Per Serving
- Calories: 102
- Saturated Fat: 0.497 gram
- Monounsaturated Fat: 1.327 grams
- Polyunsaturated Fat: 1.615 grams
- Total Fat: 3.586 grams
- Percentage of Calories From Fat: 30%

A favorite in all Arab countries, hummus is also served in Greece, Turkey and Israel. It goes well with whole-wheat pita bread cut into pie-shaped pieces or with any crunchy vegetable. Chickpeas are not only healthy but satisfying when hunger strikes.

½   cup canned chickpeas, or garbanzo beans, drained (save the liquid)
1   tsp. sesame oil (or olive oil, if preferred)
2   cloves (or less) garlic
3–4 tbsp. lemon juice
    Dash of salt
    Dash of ground cumin
    Dash of paprika (or cayenne pepper, if preferred)
    Chopped fresh parsley or dill for garnish (if desired)

1. Using a blender or food processor mix 2 to 3 tablespoons of the chickpea liquid and the oil, garlic and 2 tablespoons of the lemon juice. Blend until smooth.
2. Add the chickpeas and blend again until smooth. If necessary for a thinner consistency, use more of the lemon juice.
3. Season the mixture with the salt and more of the lemon juice to taste. Add the cumin. Sprinkle with the paprika or cayenne pepper. Decorate with the parsley or dill if using. The dip will keep for days if refrigerated. Serve it at room temperature, as the Turks do.

FRANCE

BOURSIN (SPICED CHEESE)

Nutrition Facts
Number of Servings: 2
Per Serving
- Calories: 125
- Saturated Fat: 0.025 gram
- Monounsaturated Fat: 0.012 gram
- Polyunsaturated Fat: 0.006 gram
- Total Fat: 3.108 grams
- Percentage of Calories From Fat: 25%

If you coat this cheese with grape seeds, you are truly French. It can also be coated with herbs. Here I have used cracked pepper to infuse the cheese with aroma. Serve with crisp vegetable dippers.

2/3	cup low-fat ricotta cheese
1/2	tsp. garlic powder
1	tbsp. chopped dried chives
1/2	tsp. onion powder
2	tsp. minced dried parsley
2	tbsp. instant nonfat dry milk
2	dashes crumbled dried thyme
2	tbsp. fat-free mayonnaise
	Salt
	Cracked pepper

1. With a rotary beater cream the cheese until smooth. Stir in the remaining ingredients except the cracked pepper, adding the salt to taste. Form into a patty. Wrap and chill overnight.
2. Pick up the patty with a spatula and roll it in the cracked pepper, molding the patty into a small brick. Refrigerate until hardened and ready to serve.

Note: In this recipe it is best to use only dried herbs and spices for consistency.

SMOKED OYSTER DIP

Nutrition Facts
Number of Servings: 4
Per Serving
- Calories: 55
- Saturated Fat: 0.138 gram
- Monounsaturated Fat: 0.058 gram
- Polyunsaturated Fat: 0.204 gram
- Total Fat: 1.147 grams
- Percentage of Calories From Fat: 19%

A last-minute impromptu! Quick to make.

1/3 cup low-fat ricotta cheese or low-fat creamed
    cottage cheese
2   tbsp. fat-free mayonnaise
2   tbsp. lemon juice
1   tbsp. pimiento juice
1   tbsp. minced green onions
1   tsp. chopped canned pimientos
    Dash of freshly ground pepper
1   can (3 1/2 oz.) smoked oysters, drained and
    chopped
    Lemon slices for garnish

1. In a blender jar whirl the first 5 ingredients until
   smooth.
2. Arrange in a serving bowl and add the pimientos,
   pepper and oysters. Surround with the lemon slices.
3. Serve cold with any crunchy vegetable dipper.

MUSHROOMS STUFFED WITH CRAB

Nutrition Facts
  Number of Servings: 6
  Per Serving
  • Calories: 66
  • Saturated Fat: 0.182 gram
  • Monounsaturated Fat: 0.144 gram
  • Polyunsaturated Fat: 0.588 gram
  • Total Fat: 1.132 grams
  • Percentage of Calories From Fat: 14%

When these two culinary aristocrats come together, we can have the best with less (fat).

24 (or more, depending on size) large mushrooms
      Garlic powder
1   6 ½-oz. can crabmeat, drained
6   tbsp. low-fat mayonnaise
1   tsp. minced fresh parsley
1   tbsp. minced fresh tarragon or 1 tsp. dried tarragon
1   tsp. prepared Dijon or other strong mustard
1   tsp. instant nonfat dry milk
1   tbsp. minced pimientos
      Salt
      Freshly ground pepper
      Lemon juice

1. Wash the mushrooms and dry with paper towels. Delicately cut off the stems (save them for soup).
2. Dust the mushroom hollows with the garlic powder. In a bowl mix the remaining ingredients except the pepper and lemon juice, adding the salt to taste, and fill the shells.
3. Lightly coat a baking sheet or pan with olive oil spray and arrange the mushrooms on it. Bake at 375° until hot.
4. Dust with the pepper and drizzle with the lemon juice.

TURNIPS
À LA LEBANESE

Nutrition Facts
  Number of Servings: 4
  Per Serving
  • Calories: 50
  • Saturated Fat: 0.161 gram
  • Monounsaturated Fat: 0.83 gram
  • Polyunsaturated Fat: 0.137 gram
  • Total Fat: 1.236 grams
  • Percentage of Calories From Fat: 30%

A pickled appetizer from an exotic country. It works with jicama as well and is a refreshing change from the plain carrot stick.

1	lb. raw turnips
	Red wine vinegar
2	whole cloves
	Pinch of ground cumin
1	tsp. salt
	Beet juice (save the beets for soup or salad)
1	tsp. olive oil

1. Peel the turnips and cut into sticks the size of thin french fries. Arrange in a large glass dish and pour in just enough vinegar to cover the turnips.
2. Drain the vinegar into a small saucepan with the cloves and cumin. Bring to a boil for a minute or so to reduce tartness.
3. Sprinkle the turnips evenly with the salt. Add the boiled vinegar and enough of the beet juice to color.
4. Cover and marinate overnight, turning occasionally. Drain and eat cold, drizzled with the oil.

ATHENIAN EGGPLANT

Nutrition Facts

Number of Servings: 4

Per Serving
- Calories: 75
- Saturated Fat: 0.375 gram
- Monounsaturated Fat: 1.679 grams
- Polyunsaturated Fat: 0.308 gram
- Total Fat: 2.591 grams
- Percentage of Calories From Fat: 28%

In one form or another the eggplant appears in Greek traditional meals. It is served as either a salad or an appetizer. This favorite of mine is always welcome as a dip to be scooped up with pita bread or a grape or cabbage leaf.

2	medium eggplants
	Juice of 2 lemons
8	cloves garlic, pureed
1/4	cup nonfat yogurt
1	tsp. crumbled oregano
1/4	tsp. crumbled dried basil
1	tbsp. minced fresh dill or 1 tsp. dried dill
2	tsp. olive oil
	Parsley
	Salt and freshly ground pepper

1. Preheat the broiler. Put the unpeeled eggplants on the broiler rack and turn them often, so the peels char all over. Watch them so that they do not explode.
2. Place them in a bowl and, when cool enough, remove and discard the peels and seeds. Chop the pulp, adding the lemon juice as you do to prevent darkening. The eggplant flesh will be a lovely white color.
3. In a blender jar combine the eggplant, garlic, yogurt, oregano, basil, dill, oil and parsley to taste and whirl until smooth. Add the salt and pepper to taste. This can be prepared days ahead and refrigerated. Eat at room temperature or chilled.

A Tip for the Cook

Here's what those terms on the European olive oil labels mean:

Virgin—Pressed (not chemically extracted) from the fruit and pit. In U.S.-produced oils, it means the first pressing.

Extra-Virgin—The top-quality oil from the first pressing. It must have an acidity level of less than 1 percent.

Pure—Refined and filtered to reduce acidity and lighten color and aroma. It will have a less "olivey" taste.

Refined—Second-pressed and chemically refined oil. This is a U.S. term.

Extra-Light—Extra-refined to give it a pale color and mild flavor. Not light in fat or calories.

ARTICHOKES VINAIGRETTE

Nutrition Facts
Number of Servings: 4
Per Serving
- Calories: 96
- Saturated Fat: 0.064 gram
- Monounsaturated Fat: 0.013 gram
- Polyunsaturated Fat: 0.124 gram
- Total Fat: 0.37 gram
- Percentage of Calories From Fat: 3%

A tradition in France and Belgium, this is a satisfying appetizer that will keep you nibbling.

4	medium artichokes
8	tbsp. fat-free mayonnaise
3	tbsp. white vinegar
4	tbsp. chopped fresh chives
2	cloves garlic, minced
1	tsp. prepared mustard
4	tbsp. lemon juice
1 1/2	tsp. crushed oregano leaves
1	tbsp. minced capers (if desired but preferable)
	Pinch of minced fresh tarragon

1. Wash the artichokes under running water. With a sharp knife cut off the tips.
2. Drop the artichokes into boiling salted water and cover. Simmer until the outer leaves pull off easily, about 40 minutes. Or use a pressure cooker with 1 cup boiling water for 6 to 12 minutes after the timer control moves continuously.
3. Turn the artichokes upside down in a colander to drain. Keep warm.
4. Combine the remaining ingredients and divide evenly into 4 small individual custard cups or small bowls. Serve the artichokes on individual plates with their sauce dishes.
5. To eat, pull 1 leaf at a time and dip the meaty part of the leaf into the sauce and scrape off between your teeth. The prize is the heart as well as the stem. But don't forget to remove the fuzzy portion, which is inedible.

YOGURT DRINK

Nutrition Facts
  Number of Servings: 1
  Per Serving
  • Calories: 112
  • Saturated Fat: 0.079 gram
  • Monounsaturated Fat: 0.034 gram
  • Polyunsaturated Fat: 0.004 gram
  • Total Fat: 0.147 gram
  • Percentage of Calories From Fat: 1%

When it comes to yogurt, a new healthy habit is sweeping the United States: drinkable yogurt. In India it is an old tradition, flavored with rosewater and garnished with sprigs of fresh, aromatic mint. The rosewater can be found in gourmet departments of supermarkets as well as in Greek and Middle and Far Eastern shops.

  ½   cup low-fat yogurt, thinned with ½ cup water
  ½   tsp. rosewater
  1   tbsp. sugar or honey (or grenadine or raspberry
      syrup if available)
      Drop of red food coloring (if desired and if no
      syrup was used)
  4   ice cubes, cracked
      Sprig of fresh mint, minced, or crumbled dried
      mint

1. In a blender jar combine all of the ingredients except the mint. Blend just until the ice is crushed.
2. Pour into an elegant stem glass and top with the mint. This is most cooling when sipped with a straw.

PIÑA COLADA

Nutrition Facts
Number of Servings: 1
Per Serving
- Calories: 276
- Saturated Fat: 0.319 gram
- Monounsaturated Fat: 0.147 gram
- Polyunsaturated Fat: 0.066 gram
- Total Fat: 0.643 gram
- Percentage of Calories From Fat: 2%

If you own a juicer (not essential), this drink will become a frothy nectar so rich in texture and flavor that only one glass will last for a whole happy hour.

½	cup canned crushed pineapple in its own juice, frozen solid, or ½ whole pineapple, cored and pressed through a juicer
¾	cup evaporated skim milk
¼	tsp. coconut flavoring
1	tbsp. raw sugar
	Pinch of powdered ginger
¼–½ tsp.	rum flavoring
	Pinch of ground nutmeg or mace

1. In a blender jar combine all of the ingredients except the nutmeg or mace. Blend at high speed until just creamy and foamy. (If using a juicer, add all of the ingredients except the nutmeg or mace to the pineapple juice and mix well.)
2. Pour into a glass and sprinkle the foam with the nutmeg or mace.

FETTUCCINE CON PESTO

Nutrition Facts
Number of Servings: 4
Per Serving
- Calories: 336
- Saturated Fat: 2.5 grams
- Monounsaturated Fat: 5.907 grams
- Polyunsaturated Fat: 1.829 grams
- Total Fat: 11.43 grams
- Percentage of Calories From Fat: 30%

A nonmeat dish that is so complete you may want to make it your main dish.

1	cup fresh basil leaves
2	tbsp. olive oil
8	tbsp. drained and pureed canned chickpeas, or garbanzo beans
1/4	cup grated Parmesan cheese
1	tbsp. pine nuts
1 1/2	tsp. minced garlic
1/4	tsp. salt
1/4	tsp. freshly ground pepper
2	cups fettuccine, cooked al dente in boiling salted water and kept warm (save the liquid)

1. In a blender jar combine the basil, oil, chickpea puree, cheese, pine nuts, garlic, salt and pepper. Whirl until smooth, adding 2 tablespoons or more of the salted water if the consistency is too thick. It should resemble a thick puree but remain pourable.
2. Pour over the warm fettuccine. Toss the pasta with the pesto and serve at once.

SOUPS

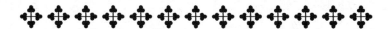

M ost soups have few calories. The ones I have chosen to "decalorize" have rich textures and satisfying tastes, and you can hardly tell them apart from their fattier sisters.

Soups are traditional in Europe. There is no meal that starts without a soup. If eaten at night, the soup is the meal, it is so complete.

Often children who hate vegetables will gulp down their entire daily quota of vegetables in one succulent bowl of soup.

Soups are elegant and filling. They are replete with minerals and vitamins and are the greatest aid to those of us who need that feeling of fullness. Can you visualize a cold winter night without the comfort of a bubbling, hot soup? I cannot.

When it comes to soups, a blender or food processor is magical! It takes minutes to convert any fresh or left-over vegetable in your refrigerator into a mouthwatering potage.

Soups have a dual purpose: to keep you trim and to keep you healthy!

CREAM OF SPINACH SOUP

Nutrition Facts
  Number of Servings: 1
  Per Serving
  • Calories: 283
  • Saturated Fat: 1.577 grams
  • Monounsaturated Fat: 6.879 grams
  • Polyunsaturated Fat: 0.998 gram
  • Total Fat: 10.29 grams
  • Percentage of Calories From Fat: 30%

"Eat your spinach!" Sound familiar?
  With this version you will need no coaxing. It's thick and delicious and so healthy.

1	large bunch parsley
1/2	cup evaporated skim milk (or buttermilk, if preferred)
1	cup cooked spinach, well drained
1/8	tsp. ground nutmeg
2	tbsp. (or more) lemon juice
1	chicken bouillon cube
1	tbsp. finely chopped fresh onions
2	tsp. olive oil
3	small leaves fresh mint or 1/4 tsp. dried mint

1. Discard the parsley stems and chop the parsley. In a saucepan combine the parsley with 1/4 cup water and a dash of salt. Simmer until soft. Drain well.
2. In a blender jar combine the remaining ingredients, starting with the milk or buttermilk. Blend until smooth. If it's too thick, add water, 1/4 cup at a time, until it's the desired consistency. Add the softened parsley.
3. Serve hot or cold.

CORN SOUP

Nutrition Facts
  Number of Servings: 4
  Per Serving
  • Calories: 184
  • Saturated Fat: 0.788 gram
  • Monounsaturated Fat: 0.649 gram
  • Polyunsaturated Fat: 1.042 grams
  • Total Fat: 3.401 grams
  • Percentage of Calories From Fat: 15%

Keep your guests guessing. Once they taste this soup, be ready to hand out the recipe. This is pure velveteen sliding over your tongue.

1   cup evaporated skim milk
1   16-oz. can corn, cooked and drained (save the liquid)
2   chicken bouillon cubes
    Dash of freshly ground pepper
1   egg, separated
2   thin slices low-fat or fat-free ham
4   tbsp. minced green onions
2   tsp. sesame seeds

1. In a blender jar, starting with the milk, combine the milk, corn, bouillon and pepper and blend for several minutes until completely smooth and creamy. If necessary, add some of the corn liquid to thin. Pour the soup into a small saucepan and simmer.
2. Beat the egg white until stiff peaks form. With a fork beat the egg yolk into the heated soup. It will form strings. Fold in the beaten egg whites. Allow this mixture to barely simmer until the egg is cooked. Do not let it boil.
3. Slice the ham into extremely thin strips and garnish the top of the soup. Sprinkle with the onions and sesame seeds.

VELOUTÉ DE CRESSON (CREAM OF WATERCRESS)

Nutrition Facts
Number of Servings: 2
Per Serving
- Calories: 316
- Saturated Fat: 7.393 grams
- Monounsaturated Fat: 3.418 grams
- Polyunsaturated Fat: 0.515 gram
- Total Fat: 11.96 grams
- Percentage of Calories From Fat: 33%

Cold or warm, this soup remains elegant and filled with vitamins. A much-asked-for recipe.

2	large bunches fresh watercress
1	large stalk celery
1	tbsp. minced onions
1	cup evaporated skim milk
1	cup diced cooked potatoes
1	tsp. bouillon powder
2	tbsp. butter or 2 tbsp. olive oil if served cold
	Salt and freshly ground pepper
	Pinch of fresh dill
	Sprig of cilantro or parsley for garnish

1. Put 1 cup water in a saucepan and add the watercress, celery and onions. Cover and simmer until the watercress is wilted but still green. Drain but save the liquid.
2. In a blender jar, starting with the milk, combine the milk, potatoes, bouillon and butter or olive oil and blend until smooth. If the soup is too thick, add the reserved liquid, 1/4 cup at a time. Season with the salt and pepper.
3. Serve hot or cold, dusted with the dill and garnished with the cilantro or parsley.

POTAGE JULIENNE

Nutrition Facts

Number of Servings: 3

Per Serving

- Calories: 140
- Saturated Fat: 2.461 grams
- Monounsaturated Fat: 1.159 grams
- Polyunsaturated Fat: 0.313 gram
- Total Fat: 4.432 grams
- Percentage of Calories From Fat: 27%

This soup is like a bouquet of vegetables, crunchy and rich. After I served this soup at a small dinner party here in Mexico, my phone did not stop ringing.

1	small (2 oz.) carrot
1	small (2 oz.) raw beet
1	medium (2 oz.) parsnip
½	medium (2 oz.) onion
1	small (2 oz.) leek (white part only)
3	chicken bouillon cubes
	Salt and freshly ground pepper
4 or 5	leaves escarole or lettuce, chopped
½	cup fresh or frozen peas
	Pinch of sugar
1½	tsp. fresh dill
1	tbsp. butter or olive oil
1½	tsp. Maggi seasoning

1. Peel the carrot, beet and parsnip and cut them into thin strips. Cut the onion into thin rings and chop the leek.
2. Combine the vegetables in a kettle. Add the bouillon, 6 cups water and the salt and pepper to taste. Bring to a boil, cover and simmer until the vegetables are almost tender.
3. Add the escarole or lettuce, peas and sugar. Leave simmering, uncovered, until the liquid is somewhat reduced and the peas are soft.
4. Serve hot, dusted with the dill and dotted with the oil or butter. Add the seasoning.

ZUPPA DE ZUCCHINI

Nutrition Facts
Number of Servings: 4
Per Serving
- Calories: 104
- Saturated Fat: 1.937 grams
- Monounsaturated Fat: 0.888 gram
- Polyunsaturated Fat: 0.317 gram
- Total Fat: 3.432 grams
- Percentage of Calories From Fat: 26%

Smooth, buttery and sweet. None of your guests will know what they are eating, but they will ask for "encores."

2 large unpeeled zucchini, thickly sliced
1/2 cup evaporated skim milk
2 cloves garlic, minced
1 vegetable bouillon cube
Salt and freshly ground pepper
1 tbsp. butter or olive oil
Pinch of dried tarragon

1. Put the zucchini in 2 cups boiling water and simmer, covered, until the zucchini is tender. Drain but save the liquid.
2. In a blender jar, starting with the milk, combine the milk, garlic, bouillion and cooked zucchini. Blend until smooth, adding the reserved liquid, 1/2 cup at a time, until the desired consistency is reached. Add the salt and pepper to taste.
3. Serve hot, dotted with the butter or oil. Dust with the tarragon.

VICHYSSOISE

Nutrition Facts
Number of Servings: 1
Per Serving
- Calories: 531
- Saturated Fat: 7.564 grams
- Monounsaturated Fat: 3.483 grams
- Polyunsaturated Fat: 0.93 gram
- Total Fat: 12.85 grams
- Percentage of Calories From Fat: 21%

A legendary rich soup. Now you can indulge, and it takes only minutes to make. If served cold, this soup looks dazzling in long-stemmed glasses.

1	medium (about 3 oz.) potato, diced
2	oz. chopped onions
2	oz. chopped leeks
1	tsp. chicken seasoning
	Salt and freshly ground pepper
1	tbsp. minced fresh parsley
1	tbsp. butter
	Pinch of fresh dill
3/4	cup evaporated skim milk
	Sprig of cilantro or parsley for garnish (if desired)

1. In a medium skillet combine the first 4 ingredients with 1 cup water. Cook slowly, covered, for about 12 to 15 minutes, or until the vegetables are tender. The liquid should be somewhat reduced.
2. Add the salt and pepper to taste, parsley, butter and dill. In a blender jar, starting with the milk, combine the milk and vegetable mixture and blend until creamy.
3. Eat chilled or warm. Garnish with the cilantro or parsley if using.

VELOUTÉ DE POIS (CREAM OF PEA)

Nutrition Facts
  Number of Servings: 4
  Per Serving
  • Calories: 152
  • Saturated Fat: 2.52 grams
  • Monounsaturated Fat: 1.174 grams
  • Polyunsaturated Fat: 0.265 gram
  • Total Fat: 4.283 grams
  • Percentage of Calories From Fat: 25%

The difference between cream of pea soup and this one is the same as the difference between corduroy and velvet. At the start of a meal this velouté will smooth the road.

1 ½   cups fresh or frozen peas
  ¼   head or 1 heart iceberg lettuce, chopped
  ⅔   cup chopped onions
  2   chicken bouillon cubes
  ¼   tsp. dried tarragon
  1   cup evaporated skim milk
  4   tsp. butter
      Salt and freshly ground pepper
  8   leaves mint, chopped, or ¼ tsp. crumbled dried mint

1. In a saucepan combine the peas, lettuce, onions, bouillon and ½ cup water. Cover and simmer until the peas are tender but still green.
2. In a blender jar combine the mixture with the tarragon, milk, butter and salt and pepper to taste. Whirl until smooth.
3. Pour into serving bowls, sprinkle with the mint and chill.

CUCUMBER SOUP

Nutrition Facts
Number of Servings: 4
Per Serving
- Calories: 91
- Saturated Fat: 0.26 gram
- Monounsaturated Fat: 0.227 gram
- Polyunsaturated Fat: 0.332 gram
- Total Fat: 1.059 grams
- Percentage of Calories From Fat: 9%

This low-key but refreshing soup hardly bites into your calorie count.

4　medium cucumbers, peeled
2–3　leeks, chopped (white part only)
　　Salt and freshly ground white pepper
2　slices whole-grain bread
　　Dash of ground nutmeg
4　sprigs fresh parsley or 2 tsp. dried parsley
2　tsp. lemon juice
　　Thin slices of cucumber or sprigs of parsley,
　　cilantro or dill for garnish

1. Cut the cucumbers lengthwise into sticks, removing the seeds. Cube into bite-size pieces.
2. Place the cucumbers in a saucepan and cover with water; add the leeks and salt and pepper to taste. Simmer, covered, for 15 to 20 minutes.
3. Remove the vegetables with a slotted spoon and keep warm. Pour the remaining liquid into a blender jar and add the bread, nutmeg and parsley. Blend until smooth.
4. Pour into a small skillet over medium heat and cook, stirring, until thickened. Add the warm vegetables, lemon juice and more of the salt and pepper to taste. Serve warm with the cucumbers, parsley, cilantro or dill for garnish.

AVGOLEMONO CHICKEN RICE SOUP

Nutrition Facts
  Number of Servings: 1
  Per Serving
  • Calories: 488
  • Saturated Fat: 5.333 grams
  • Monounsaturated Fat: 4.807 grams
  • Polyunsaturated Fat: 2.133 grams
  • Total Fat: 14.08 grams
  • Percentage of Calories From Fat: 26%

A traditional Greek soup filled with health. I have given the recipe for one portion, but I can never finish it in one sitting. Why not apportion it for one dinner and luncheon?

4	oz. boneless, skinless chicken breast
1	chicken bouillon cube
1/4	cup sliced carrots
6	very thin slices onion
1	stalk celery, finely diced
1	tbsp. chopped fresh parsley
1/4	tsp. crumbled oregano
1	clove garlic, minced
	Salt
3	tbsp. uncooked brown rice
	Freshly ground pepper
1	large egg, separated
	Juice of 1 lemon
1	tsp. butter or olive oil

1. In a saucepan combine the chicken, 2 cups water, bouillon, carrots, onions, celery, parsley, oregano, garlic and 1/4 teaspoon of the salt. Cover and simmer for 15 to 20 minutes.
2. Add the rice, increase the heat and bring to a boil. Cover and simmer for another 30 minutes, or until the chicken is tender; add the pepper and more of the salt to taste.
3. Remove the chicken, chop it into bite-size pieces and return it to the soup. Increase the heat and cook the broth, uncovered, until it is reduced to about 1 cup liquid.
4. At serving time beat the egg white until stiff. Beat in the yolk and then the lemon juice. Pour the egg mixture on top of the warm soup. Cover the pot and barely simmer until the egg is cooked. The egg will curdle a bit.
5. When the soup is hot and slightly thickened, serve dotted with the butter or oil.

NEW YORK CLAM CHOWDER

Nutrition Facts
Number of Servings: 1
Per Serving
- Calories: 447
- Saturated Fat: 2.717 grams
- Monounsaturated Fat: 10.15 grams
- Polyunsaturated Fat: 2.218 grams
- Total Fat: 18 grams
- Percentage of Calories From Fat: 31%

Americans know that a good New York clam chowder is a whole meal in itself. This low-fat, "decalorized" version is no different.

6	oz. clams, chopped (save the liquid)
1/2	cup diced carrots
1/4	cup coarsely chopped onions
1 1/2	stalks celery, chopped
1	chicken bouillon cube
3/4	cup tomato juice
3/4	cup tomato sauce
1/2	cup fresh green beans, cut into pieces
1	medium yellow summer squash, cut into pieces
3	tbsp. chopped fresh parsley or 1 tbsp. dried parsley
	Worcestershire sauce
	Salt and freshly ground pepper
1	tbsp. olive oil

1. In a saucepan combine the clam liquid, carrots, onions, celery, bouillon and 1/4 cup water. Cover and simmer for 15 minutes, adding more water if necessary, until the vegetables are tender and the liquid is absorbed.
2. Add the tomato juice, tomato sauce, beans and squash. Cover and simmer for 15 minutes, or until the beans are tender but still firm.
3. Add the clams, parsley and Worcestershire sauce and salt and pepper to taste. Heat and serve, drizzled with the oil.

OYSTER SOUP WITH CROUTONS

Nutrition Facts
Number of Servings: 2
Per Serving
- Calories: 306
- Saturated Fat: 1.475 grams
- Monounsaturated Fat: 0.924 gram
- Polyunsaturated Fat: 1.555 grams
- Total Fat: 5.617 grams
- Percentage of Calories From Fat: 17%

It is so rich that it could be called an oyster stew!

2	slices multigrain bread
	Powdered thyme
	Garlic powder
12	oz. fresh cooked or canned oysters (save the liquid)
3	stalks celery, finely chopped
2	small cloves garlic, minced
1	cup evaporated skim milk
1	chicken bouillon cube
1/4	tsp. onion powder
1/4	tsp. crumbled dried tarragon
1	tbsp. minced fresh parsley or 1 tsp. dried parsley
	Salt and freshly ground pepper
2	thin slices lime for garnish

1. Make the croutons by cutting the bread into cubes and dusting them lightly with thyme and garlic powder. Place on a baking sheet and bake at 300° until they begin to brown. Reserve on a rack to dry.
2. In a saucepan combine the oyster liquid, celery and garlic. Simmer, adding water as necessary if the oyster liquid evaporates, until the celery is tender but firm.
3. Add the oysters, milk, bouillon, onion powder, tarragon, parsley and half of the croutons. Heat very slowly, stirring (do not let it simmer). Add the salt and pepper to taste.
4. Pour into serving bowls and top with the remaining croutons and the lime slices.

CREAM OF MUSHROOM SOUP

Nutrition Facts
  Number of Servings: 1
  Per Serving
  • Calories: 168
  • Saturated Fat: 2.669 grams
  • Monounsaturated Fat: 1.216 grams
  • Polyunsaturated Fat: 0.277 gram
  • Total Fat: 4.528 grams
  • Percentage of Calories From Fat: 24%

Filling and creamy—while making no demands on your calorie count.

1	cup sliced fresh mushrooms
1	chicken bouillon cube
1/4	tsp. onion powder
1	tbsp. minced fresh parsley or 1 tsp. dried parsley
	Salt and freshly ground pepper
	Pinch of ground nutmeg
1/2	cup evaporated skim milk
1/2	tsp. chopped fresh dill or pinch of dried dill
1	tsp. butter

1. Combine the mushrooms, bouillon, onion powder, parsley and 1 cup water in a saucepan. Simmer, uncovered, until the liquid is reduced to 1/2 cup.
2. Pour this into a blender jar. Add the salt and pepper to taste and the nutmeg and blend until creamy.
3. Return to the pan and add the milk. Heat to serving temperature.
4. Sprinkle with the dill and top with the butter. Eat warm.

COLD BORSCHT

Nutrition Facts
  Number of Servings: 1
  Per Serving
  • Calories: 158
  • Saturated Fat: 0.384 gram
  • Monounsaturated Fat: 0.196 gram
  • Polyunsaturated Fat: 0.139 gram
  • Total Fat: 0.849 gram
  • Percentage of Calories From Fat: 4%

Rich and red in color. Refreshing on those hot summer days. Quick and easy to assemble, too.

½ cup cooked sliced beets, drained (save 3–6 tbsp. of the liquid)
¼ cup cooked sliced carrots, drained
¼ cup tomato puree
¼ cup buttermilk or low-fat yogurt
1 clove garlic, minced
1 beef bouillon cube
2 tbsp. lemon or lime juice
   Salt and freshly ground pepper
   Dill
   Fresh mint

1. In a blender jar combine the first 7 ingredients. Add about 3 tablespoons of the beet liquid. Whirl until creamy and smooth.
2. Add more of the beet liquid, 1 spoonful at a time, if necessary for a creamy consistency. Add the salt and pepper to taste.
3. Chill thoroughly. Top with the dill and mint.

CONSOMMÉ MADRILENE EN GELÉE

Nutrition Facts
Number of Servings: 3
Per Serving
- Calories: 102
- Saturated Fat: 0.022 gram
- Monounsaturated Fat: 0.022 gram
- Polyunsaturated Fat: 0.057 gram
- Total Fat: 0.164 gram
- Percentage of Calories From Fat: 1%

Serve cold in oversize wine goblets.

1½ envelopes unflavored gelatin
2 cups tomato juice (shake the container well before pouring)
½ tsp. Worcestershire sauce
2 beef bouillon cubes
¼ tsp. onion powder
2 tsp. balsamic or red wine vinegar
Juice of 2 limes
Salt and freshly ground pepper
Rind of 1 lime, finely grated
6 ice cubes, cracked
1 tsp. black caviar for garnish
Sprigs of parsley or cilantro for garnish

1. In a saucepan let the gelatin soften in the tomato juice. Heat and stir constantly until the gelatin is dissolved.
2. Add the Worcestershire sauce, bouillon, onion powder, vinegar and lime juice; heat until the bouillon is dissolved. Add the salt and pepper to taste.
3. Pour into a bowl and chill until set. Then put the mixture in a blender jar and whirl, adding the lime rind and cracked ice a bit at a time until the mixture has doubled in volume and is a pale pink color.
4. Garnish with the caviar and parsley or cilantro.

SOUPE À L'OIGNON AU GRATIN

Nutrition Facts
  Number of Servings: 1
  Per Serving
  • Calories: 296
  • Saturated Fat: 5.766 grams
  • Monounsaturated Fat: 3.836 grams
  • Polyunsaturated Fat: 0.431 gram
  • Total Fat: 11.7 grams
  • Percentage of Calories From Fat: 35%

A legend all its own, yet so simple to prepare.

1	medium (4 oz.) onion, thinly sliced
½	tsp. onion powder
1	beef bouillon cube
	Salt and freshly ground pepper
1	slice whole-wheat bread, toasted until crisp
½	cup shredded low-fat Swiss cheese
1	tbsp. grated Parmesan cheese

1. Preheat the oven to 350°.
2. Coat a nonstick skillet with olive oil spray and sauté the onions until wilted. Add 1¼ cups water to the skillet and bring to a quick boil. Add the onion powder, bouillon and salt and pepper to taste; stir to dissolve the bouillon.
3. Pour the soup into an ovenproof earthenware ramekin. Slightly immerse the bread on top of the soup. Place the Swiss cheese on the bread and cover with the Parmesan. Add more of the pepper to taste.
4. Place the dish in the oven. Bake for 10 minutes, or until the top is browned and the cheese is bubbly.

NEW ENGLAND CLAM CHOWDER

Nutrition Facts
  Number of Servings: 1
  Per Serving
  • Calories: 370
  • Saturated Fat: 3.186 grams
  • Monounsaturated Fat: 3.75 grams
  • Polyunsaturated Fat: 1.274 grams
  • Total Fat: 8.541 grams
  • Percentage of Calories From Fat: 20%

There is no American tradition without apple pie and New England clam chowder! The rich and creamy taste belies the calories.

1	tsp. chicken seasoning
¼	cup chopped scallions
1	medium (3 oz.) potato, diced
¼	cup diced carrots
2	tsp. low-fat or fat-free margarine
2	tsp. arrowroot
¾	cup evaporated skim milk
½	cup canned clams, drained and minced (save ¼–½ cup of the liquid)
	Salt and freshly ground pepper
	Minced fresh parsley for garnish
	Pinch of ground nutmeg or mace for garnish
1	tbsp. butter

1. In a medium skillet combine 1 cup water and the chicken seasoning, scallions, potatoes and carrots. Bring to a boil and simmer until the vegetables are tender, about 15 minutes. Reserve the vegetables and ½ cup of the pan liquid.
2. In a small skillet melt the margarine and sprinkle with the arrowroot to make a paste. Over medium heat add the milk, slowly stirring constantly until smooth and thickened.
3. Add the reserved vegetables and pan liquid, the clams, some of the clam liquid and salt and pepper to taste. Cook, stirring and adding more of the clam liquid if too thick.
4. Serve piping hot, garnished with the parsley and nutmeg or mace. Drizzle with the butter.

A TIP FOR THE COOK

If any of your soup recipes call for heavy cream to thicken them, use evaporated skim milk instead. You'll get the same rich body with hardly any fat. If the recipe calls for whole milk, use nonfat or skim milk to which you've added a tablespoon of instant nonfat dry milk per cup as a thickener.

GAZPACHO

Nutrition Facts
  Number of Servings: 4
  Per Serving
  • Calories: 135
  • Saturated Fat: 0.2 gram
  • Monounsaturated Fat: 0.276 gram
  • Polyunsaturated Fat: 0.554 gram
  • Total Fat: 1.8 grams
  • Percentage of Calories From Fat: 11%

A cold gazpacho is refreshing as a liquid salad or a chunky soup. Either one will set the pace for the unusual. It is not only colorful but a bowlful of vitamins, too.

4   medium tomatoes, peeled and cubed
4   medium cloves garlic
1   medium (5 oz.) onion
1   tsp. chicken bouillon
    Salt and freshly ground pepper
1   medium cucumber, diced
1   sweet red bell pepper, diced very small
1   medium green pepper, diced very small
4   slices whole-wheat bread, toasted, dried and cubed

1. In a blender jar combine the tomatoes, garlic, onion and bouillon. Blend until smooth, adding water if necessary. The mixture should be thick.
2. Season with the salt and ground pepper. Pour into 4 soup bowls and chill thoroughly.
3. When ready to serve, top each bowl with a quarter of the cucumbers, red and green peppers and bread cubes. Eat immediately.

MAIN-DISH
SALADS

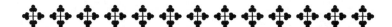

"I am sick of lettuce!" the people in my classes would say. I would ask, "How do you fix your lettuce leaves?"

And together we would begin to imagine what it is like to be lettuce, naked and simple. How we could dress it up and take it places. How we could accommodate it in a thousand different ways.

By the time the classes ended, each of my students had found a new dressing, a unique approach. Then we would learn how to "decalorize" each delicacy. The results were mouthwatering salads and complete meals for the most ravenous of us.

When I served my chicken salad in a pineapple shell (recipe on page 48) here in Mexico, my new friends thought I had just graduated from culinary school! It does not take a special artist to paint with lettuce. Only imagination.

The freshness and variety of your greens are essential, as they are the basic ingredients. Wash them thoroughly and spin them dry in your salad spinner. Put them in a plastic bag and leave them in the refrigerator until ready to use. It is easier to prepare quantities ahead of time, so you can improvise at the last minute.

The greener your greens are, the healthier. Add color, and you have a palette. Add fresh herbs and spices and a pleasing dressing, and you will be crunching your vitamins and fiber with enthusiasm. And that is only the beginning…I promise.

ASPIC DE CRABE

Nutrition Facts
Number of Servings: 2
Per Serving
- Calories: 264
- Saturated Fat: 0.791 gram
- Monounsaturated Fat: 1.069 grams
- Polyunsaturated Fat: 2.424 grams
- Total Fat: 4.836 grams
- Percentage of Calories From Fat: 16%

When we think of glamour, we think slim, delicate, classy, chic and stylish. This describes this elegant aspic. And look at the calories! Served over a bed of greens and colors, it becomes the most-talked-about salad.

1   envelope unflavored gelatin
1   6-oz. can crabmeat (save the liquid)
1/2 cup evaporated skim milk
1   tsp. chicken seasoning
1/4 tsp. onion powder
1   tbsp. imitation mayonnaise
2   tsp. dried tarragon or 1 tsp. balsamic vinegar with
     1/4 tsp. dried tarragon
     Grated rind and juice of 1 or more limes
3   ice cubes, cracked
2   medium dill pickles, chopped
     Salt and freshly ground pepper
     Lettuce leaves
     Pimiento strips, radishes and capers for garnish (if desired)

1. In a bowl soften the gelatin in ¼ cup of the crabmeat liquid. Then mix with the milk, chicken seasoning and onion powder and pour into a small saucepan. Cook over low heat, stirring, until the gelatin is dissolved.
2. In a blender jar combine the gelatin mixture, mayonnaise, tarragon or vinegar, lime rind and juice and ice and whirl until the ice is dissolved. Pour into a mixing bowl and add the crabmeat with the remaining crabmeat liquid and the pickles. Mix well and add the salt and pepper to taste. Pour this into individual custard cups and chill until firm, about 2 hours.
3. When ready to serve, dip each cup in a little warm water and unmold onto a bed of the lettuce. Garnish with the pimientos, radishes and capers if using.

A Tip for the Cook

Here are some tips for having the freshest fish possible:

- Refrigerate fish as soon as possible after buying—make the fish market your last stop.
- Don't buy fish that has a "fishy" odor—fresh fish should smell like salt water.
- Look for tight, shiny scales and bright, clear eyes on whole, fresh fish.
- Buy fillets or steaks that are moist, slightly translucent and dense, not flaky.

SALMON MOUSSE

Nutrition Facts
Number of Servings: 2
Per Serving
- Calories: 241
- Saturated Fat: 1.907 grams
- Monounsaturated Fat: 2.317 grams
- Polyunsaturated Fat: 3.708 grams
- Total Fat: 8.629 grams
- Percentage of Calories From Fat: 32%

Here is how to turn a can of salmon into a light, delicious and dazzling salad. Garnish with thin lime slices. Serve with baked crackers or thin Norwegian whole-grain wafers. Or serve on a bed of fresh watercress mixed with tidbits of other greens and reds.

1/4	cup evaporated skim milk
1	6-oz. can salmon, drained (save the liquid)
	Juice of 1 lime
1	tsp. balsamic or tarragon vinegar
1	envelope unflavored gelatin
1	envelope instant onion broth or 1 tsp. onion powder
1	tbsp. fresh chives or 1 tsp. dried chives
1/8	tsp. dried tarragon
	Salt and freshly ground pepper
1	tbsp. imitation mayonnaise
	Salad greens

1. Pour the milk into a small electric mixer bowl. Place the bowl and beaters in the freezer until crystals form in the milk.
2. Remove the visible bones from the salmon and mash it very fine.
3. In a saucepan combine the salmon liquid, lime juice, vinegar, gelatin and seasonings with 1/2 cup cold water, adding the salt and pepper to taste. Stir over low heat until the gelatin is dissolved.
4. When the milk is ready, whip it with the frozen beaters until stiff peaks form.
5. Stir the mayonnaise into the salmon.
6. Fold the gelatin mixture into the whipped milk. Quickly fold in the salmon. Pour this mousse into individual molds. Refrigerate until firm.
7. When ready to serve, dip the bottom of the mold into hot water for a few seconds and unmold onto a bed of greens of your choice.

A TIP FOR THE COOK

What to do when dinner's almost ready, but the champagne/wine isn't cold? Fill an ice bucket halfway with ice cubes, add several cups of cold water and 4 tablespoons of salt and stick the bottle inside. Fill any remaining space with cold water and let it sit for 20 minutes.

PINEAPPLE-COCONUT CHICKEN LUAU

Nutrition Facts
  Number of Servings: 4
  Per Serving
  • Calories: 788
  • Saturated Fat: 3.255 grams
  • Monounsaturated Fat: 4.211 grams
  • Polyunsaturated Fat: 9.216 grams
  • Total Fat: 18.62 grams
  • Percentage of Calories From Fat: 24%

This Hawaiian salad is eye-pleasing and stomach-filling!
Combines starch, meat and three fruits.

1	medium fresh pineapple (keep the leaves on)
1 1/2	cups uncooked very thin egg noodles, cooked al dente in boiling salted water and well drained
2	cups diced cooked chicken
3	stalks celery, finely chopped
1	tsp. coconut flavoring (if desired)
1/4	cup low-sodium soy sauce
1/2	cup imitation mayonnaise
1 1/2	tsp. curry powder
1	tsp. minced fresh ginger or 1/2 tsp. ground ginger
1	medium banana, thinly sliced (sprinkle with lemon juice to prevent darkening) for garnish (if desired)
1	tangerine or small orange, cut into segments for garnish (if desired)

1. Cut the pineapple lengthwise into 4 parts. Remove the core and enough fruit to leave $1/2$ inch at the bottom. Discard the core, but reserve the cut-out fruit. Drain upside down on paper towels or in a colander for at least 30 minutes.
2. Put the shells and noodles in the refrigerator.
3. Cut the pineapple meat into small chunks and drain in a colander. In a mixing bowl combine the pineapple, chicken, celery and flavoring if using and chill.
4. At serving time drain off and discard the liquid from the chicken mixture. Toss with the soy sauce and mayonnaise. Season with the curry and ginger. Fill each shell with a quarter of the noodles, cover with a quarter of the chicken mixture and decorate with the bananas and tangerines or oranges if using.

A Tip for the Cook

If your salad recipe calls for a ranch dressing, mix your own by whisking $1/4$ cup of buttermilk with 1 teaspoon of Dijon mustard and minced garlic, parsley and chives to taste.

TOSSED SALADE NIÇOISE

Nutrition Facts
  Number of Servings: 2
  Per Serving
  • Calories: 494
  • Saturated Fat: 2.737 grams
  • Monounsaturated Fat: 10.72 grams
  • Polyunsaturated Fat: 2.614 grams
  • Total Fat: 17.52 grams
  • Percentage of Calories From Fat: 31%

The original version of salade niçoise is smothered with whole olives and a rich dressing that quadruples the calories of this one. However, all of the freshness, the crunchiness and the aroma are here.

1 1/4 cups diced potatoes, cooked until just tender
  2   cups fresh green beans cut into 1/2-inch pieces, cooked until just tender but firm
  2   firm tomatoes, cut into wedges
  2   tbsp. capers, drained
  2   cloves garlic, minced
      Romaine or leaf lettuce, torn into pieces
  1/4 cup thinly sliced red onions
  8   oz. white tuna, well drained
      Salt and freshly ground pepper
  1   tsp. Dijon mustard
  1/2 tsp. crumbled dried chervil
  1/2 tsp. crumbled dried tarragon
  1   tbsp. balsamic or tarragon vinegar
  2   tbsp. olive oil

1. Chill the potatoes and beans. Set aside some of the tomato wedges and capers for garnish.
2. Put some of the garlic in the palm of your hand and rub the salad bowl (preferably wooden) thoroughly. Add the lettuce, onions, tuna, potatoes and beans and the remaining tomatoes and capers. Add the salt and pepper to taste.
3. In a small bowl stir together the remaining garlic and the mustard, chervil, tarragon, vinegar and oil and pour over the salad. Toss. Garnish with the reserved tomatoes and capers.

A Tip for the Cook

To make your own low-fat Thousand Island dressing, stir 2 tablespoons of tomato paste into $1/2$ cup of nonfat yogurt or nonfat sour cream. Add $1/2$ teaspoon of lemon juice, and minced garlic, pickles, shallots and celery to taste. If you like it a little sweeter, add a small amount of sugar.

HAM ROLLS

Nutrition Facts
Number of Servings: 2
Per Serving
- Calories: 80.1
- Saturated Fat: 0.25 gram
- Monounsaturated Fat: 0.028 gram
- Polyunsaturated Fat: 0.213 gram
- Total Fat: 1.208 grams
- Percentage of Calories From Fat: 12%

During the rainy season stranded travelers would turn up at the plantation. We always had fresh or canned asparagus in our pantry and baked ham cured on the premises. For color we added a slice of papaya. I am still making this when I am really rushed!

1	cup cooked peas and carrots
2	tbsp. fat-free mayonnaise
1	tbsp. chopped fresh chives or green onion tops
1	tbsp. lemon or lime juice
	Salt and freshly ground pepper
	Curry powder
4	slices lean Virginia or boiled ham
8	spears cooked thin or baby asparagus
	Lettuce leaves or watercress sprigs (if available)
	Parsley sprigs or carrot curls for garnish

1. In a bowl mix the peas and carrots, mayonnaise, chives or onions and lemon or lime juice thoroughly; season with the salt, pepper and curry powder.
2. Distribute evenly in the center of each ham slice and add 2 of the asparagus spears. Roll the ham slices up, pressing the vegetables toward the sides to make even rolls.
3. Arrange the rolls on the lettuce or watercress. Garnish with the parsley or carrots.

INDIAN INSPIRED

SEAFOOD SALAD

Nutrition Facts
Number of Servings: 1
Per Serving
- Calories: 454
- Saturated Fat: 2.673 grams
- Monounsaturated Fat: 3.764 grams
- Polyunsaturated Fat: 9.016 grams
- Total Fat: 17.33 grams
- Percentage of Calories From Fat: 34%

In Rwanda many cultures lived side by side. One of our neighbors gave us this filling version of a cold, curried Indian seafood salad. We adopted it because it is simple, can be made in advance and looks great unmolded at a buffet table.

½   cup brown rice, cooked
4   oz. tuna or crabmeat, well drained
2   tbsp. low-fat mayonnaise
1   tbsp. lemon juice
1   tsp. chicken seasoning
¼   tsp. onion powder
¼   tsp. ground cumin
1   tsp. curry powder (or to taste)
     Freshly ground pepper
     Salad greens
1   tomato, cut into thin wedges, and 1 pimiento, cut into strips, for garnish

1. In a mixing bowl combine the rice, tuna or crabmeat, mayonnaise, lemon juice and seasonings, adding the pepper to taste. Pack the bowl firmly. Cover and chill for several hours.
2. Unmold onto a bed of the greens and garnish with the tomato wedges and pimientos.

GREEK SALAD

Nutrition Facts
Number of Servings: 4
Per Serving
- Calories: 50
- Saturated Fat: 0.598 gram
- Monounsaturated Fat: 0.969 gram
- Polyunsaturated Fat: 0.232 gram
- Total Fat: 1.711 grams
- Percentage of Calories From Fat: 35%

This salad has been adopted the world over. It is attractive, aromatic and healthy. It looks great in a glass bowl, but once the salad is eaten, don't get carried away and throw the glass bowl against the wall!

1	clove garlic, minced
2–3	Salonika peppers in brine or 1 large dill pickle, finely chopped
4	tsp. olive oil
4	tsp. good wine vinegar (preferably tarragon)
1/2	medium firm tomato
	Romaine lettuce, chicory or curly endive and iceberg lettuce, torn into pieces
1/2	unpeeled cucumber, thinly sliced
2	tsp. diced feta cheese
3/4	cup finely chopped green onions
	Several pinches of crumbled oregano
1	tbsp. minced fresh basil or mint or 1/4 tsp. crumbled dried basil or mint
	Salt and freshly ground pepper
2	hard-cooked eggs, cut as thinly as possible into wedges, for garnish (if desired)

1. Put some of the garlic in the palm of your hand and rub the serving bowl, crushing the garlic against the sides as well.
2. In a small bowl combine the remaining garlic and the Salonika peppers or pickles, oil and vinegar. Cut the tomato into small cubes. Add the tomatoes to the pepper mixture and stir to combine the ingredients.
3. In the garlic-smeared serving bowl combine the greens, cucumbers, cheese, onions, oregano and basil or mint. Chill.
4. When ready to serve, add the salt and ground pepper to taste and the dressing. Toss lightly. Garnish with the egg wedges.

A TIP FOR THE COOK

When a recipe calls for a "pinch" of an ingredient, how much does that mean? Just slightly less than $1/8$ teaspoon. Here are some other often used equivalent measures:

3 teaspoons	=	1 tablespoon
2 tablespoons	=	1 fluid ounce
4 tablespoons	=	$1/4$ cup or 2 fluid ounces
5 tablespoons + 1 teaspoon	=	$1/3$ cup

SHRIMP-STUFFED TOMATOES

Nutrition Facts
Number of Servings: 4
Per Serving
- Calories: 122
- Saturated Fat: 0.254 gram
- Monounsaturated Fat: 0.191 gram
- Polyunsaturated Fat: 0.489 gram
- Total Fat: 1.195 grams
- Percentage of Calories From Fat: 9%

Tomates aux crevettes is a Belgian tradition that uses the petites crevettes from the Belgian coast. I found a very similar dish in the United States, but it uses large shrimp cut to size and arranged on top of the tomato instead of inside. Your choice!

4	large ripe tomatoes
	Salt
	Freshly ground pepper
2	cups diced cooked shrimp (or 2 cups small pink shrimp from Ostende)
8	tbsp. fat-free mayonnaise
1/2	tsp. dried tarragon
1/4	tsp. dried thyme
1/4	tsp. curry powder (if desired)
2	tbsp. lemon or lime juice
1	tsp. minced capers or minced pickled cucumbers
8	leaves lettuce

1. Cut off the tomato tops (about 1/2 inch down) and remove most of the meat (save for soups) until only the shells remain. Sprinkle the shells with the salt and pepper to taste.
2. Lightly combine the remaining ingredients except the lettuce and divide among the tomatoes, stuffing each with the mixture. Chill the tomatoes.
3. At serving time arrange them on beds of the lettuce.

CHICKEN SALAD

Nutrition Facts
 Number of Servings: 4
 Per Serving
 • Calories: 147
 • Saturated Fat: 0.612 gram
 • Monounsaturated Fat: 0.722 gram
 • Polyunsaturated Fat: 0.51 gram
 • Total Fat: 2.203 grams
 • Percentage of Calories From Fat: 13%

Crunchy and sprouted, this salad has tang to boot!

2	cups diced cooked chicken
1/3	cup diced bamboo shoots
1	cup fresh bean sprouts
1	stalk celery, finely chopped
1/3	cup chopped green onions
2	tbsp. low-sodium soy sauce
1/4	cup red wine vinegar or balsamic vinegar
1	tbsp. minced fresh ginger or 1/4 tsp. ground ginger
1	tsp. sugar or honey
	Ground Szechuan pepper or finely crushed red pepper
1/4	cup fat-free mayonnaise
8	leaves lettuce
	Parsley for garnish
	Minced cilantro for garnish (if desired)

1. In a large bowl combine the first 5 ingredients.
2. In a skillet combine the remaining ingredients except the mayonnaise, lettuce, parsley and cilantro. Add the pepper to taste. Bring to a boil and pour over the salad; toss.
3. Add the mayonnaise and toss again. Chill.
4. Serve on the lettuce with the parsley and cilantro if using.

Main-Dish
Salads
❖

HOT LAMB SALAD

Nutrition Facts
  Number of Servings: 2
  Per Serving
  • Calories: 243
  • Saturated Fat: 2.679 grams
  • Monounsaturated Fat: 4.555 grams
  • Polyunsaturated Fat: 0.687 gram
  • Total Fat: 9.616 grams
  • Percentage of Calories From Fat: 35%

The latest style in salads today is to combine hot and cold. It creates a delicious contrast. This lamb salad is Greek inspired inasmuch as there is always some cold lamb in my refrigerator. The rest was put together with items available in my cupboard. When you prepare this dish, the whole neighborhood will come by!

3   large cloves garlic, minced
6   oz. cooked lean lamb, sliced or cubed
4   oz. red onion, sliced into thin rings
1   tbsp. low-sodium soy sauce
1/2 tsp. crumbled oregano
1/2 tsp. cumin seeds or 1/2 tsp. ground cumin
1   tbsp. olive oil
1   tbsp. balsamic or tarragon vinegar
     Juice of 1 lemon
     Freshly ground pepper

1. Lightly coat a nonstick skillet with olive oil spray. Turn the heat to high and add the garlic and lamb to sear on all sides. Make sure the garlic does not burn.
2. Toss the remaining ingredients in a large bowl, adding the pepper to taste, and arrange the searing-hot slices/cubes of lamb on top.

EGGS, CHEESES AND VEGETABLES

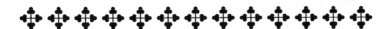

M ost health- and weight-conscious people can eat up to four eggs a week. I am one of them.

It is no secret that eggs play an important role in creative cooking. How can one have a soufflé or a quiche without an egg? Crepes, potato pancakes and eggplant parmigiana, to name a few, need eggs. Who can live without these all-time favorites?

Eggs are an excellent source of protein and are quick and easy to prepare. Calories are minimal. The egg is a good ally to any vegetable. It also replaces meat and other sources of protein. The recipes that follow—which are some of my most successful because they stretch a calorie—promote good health by including so many fresh vegetables. They are mouthwatering, satisfying meals and are particularly suited to entertaining your health-conscious friends. Virtually all of the cheeses I use are low-fat or fat-free. In goes the taste, out comes the fat!

Some of us are not allowed to eat eggs because of high cholesterol counts. Only you and your doctor know. There are excellent egg substitutes on the market, and their packages explain how to use them. Try to experiment with some of the dishes by using just egg whites, by replacing whole eggs with an egg substitute or even by adding egg whites to the egg substitute. Since my recipes are fast and simple, they are tools for experimentation and enhanced creativity.

Think about the cost of eggs versus meat!

SPINACH SOUFFLÉ

Nutrition Facts
  Number of Servings: 4
  Per Serving
  • Calories: 192
  • Saturated Fat: 3.332 grams
  • Monounsaturated Fat: 2.436 grams
  • Polyunsaturated Fat: 0.689 gram
  • Total Fat: 7.65 grams
  • Percentage of Calories From Fat: 35%

This dish will convert a spinach-hater into a spinach aficionado. It is delicious and elegant and has a low calorie count.

1	10-oz. package frozen chopped spinach, cooked
1	tbsp. cornstarch
1/2	cup evaporated skim milk
1	chicken bouillon cube
2	large eggs, separated, plus 2 additional egg whites
1/2	cup grated Parmesan cheese or Romano cheese
1/2	tsp. onion powder
1	tbsp. minced fresh garlic or 1 medium clove garlic
	Ground nutmeg
	Freshly ground pepper
1	slice whole-wheat bread, toasted, dried and blended into fine crumbs
1	tsp. imitation bacon bits
1	tsp. melted butter or olive oil

1. Drain the cooked spinach and squeeze dry.
2. Dissolve the cornstarch in the cold milk and pour into a small skillet. Cook over medium heat, stirring, until the sauce is thickened. Pour into a blender jar and add the bouillon, egg yolks, spinach, cheese, onion powder, garlic and nutmeg and pepper to taste. Blend until smooth and pour into a mixing bowl.
3. Beat the 4 egg whites until stiff but not dry. Fold the egg whites quickly but evenly into the sauce mixture.
4. Lightly coat a 4- to 6-cup soufflé dish or ramekin with olive oil spray. Pour the egg mixture into the dish. Combine the bread crumbs and bacon bits and sprinkle on the soufflé with more of the nutmeg if desired. Bake at 375° for 20 to 25 minutes, or until the center no longer wobbles when pressed with a spoon or finger. To prevent drying, do not overbake. Dot with the butter or oil.

A TIP FOR THE COOK

You can substitute beet greens in almost any recipe that calls for raw or cooked spinach. And since you get them free when you purchase beets, they can be a budget bonus. They are also a nutrition bargain, as they are full of vitamin A. Look for leaves that have a deep color and don't show signs of yellowing or wilting.

CHEESE CREPES

Nutrition Facts
Number of Servings: 1
Per Serving
- Calories: 274
- Saturated Fat: 3.837 grams
- Monounsaturated Fat: 1.649 grams
- Polyunsaturated Fat: 1.707 grams
- Total Fat: 10.38 grams
- Percentage of Calories From Fat: 33%

My daughter Tatiana's favorite! This crepe has a rich sauce teeming with mushrooms and melted cheese. Wait until you sink your teeth into this one! A whole meal.

½	cup sliced fresh mushrooms or 3 tbsp. sliced canned mushrooms
¼	cup shredded aged low-fat provolone cheese
2	tbsp. low-fat mayonnaise
1	tsp. minced fresh garlic or ⅛ tsp. garlic powder
	Salt and freshly ground pepper
1	slice multigrain or whole-wheat bread
¼	cup fat-free egg substitute
¼	cup evaporated skim milk
	Pinch of ground nutmeg

1. In a small skillet cook the fresh mushrooms in 1 tablespoon water just until limp and the water has evaporated. If using the canned mushrooms, drain and chop them.
2. In a small bowl combine the mushrooms, cheese, mayonnaise, garlic or garlic powder and salt and pepper to taste. Reserve.
3. In a blender jar combine the bread, egg substitute, milk and nutmeg. Blend until completely smooth.
4. Lightly coat a nonstick skillet with olive oil spray and preheat over medium heat. Pour in the batter, tilting the pan to spread the batter evenly. Watch the browning closely by carefully lifting the edge of the crepe with a spatula. Reduce the heat if necessary.
5. When brown flecked or evenly browned, turn the crepe. Be careful, because the crepe will tear if turned too soon. Brown the other side.
6. Spread all but 1 1/2 tablespoons of the filling over the crepe. Cover the skillet and cook over the lowest heat just until the cheese is melted.
7. Roll the crepe and spread the remaining 1 1/2 tablespoons filling over the top. Cover and heat until the cheese starts melting.

CHEDDAR-ONION PIE

Nutrition Facts
Number of Servings: 4
Per Serving
- Calories: 362
- Saturated Fat: 3.975 grams
- Monounsaturated Fat: 1.978 grams
- Polyunsaturated Fat: 0.401 gram
- Total Fat: 13.07 grams
- Percentage of Calories From Fat: 31%

An earthy, English dish the whole family will love.

4	medium onions, very thinly sliced
2	tsp. chicken seasoning
	Freshly ground pepper
1/2	cup evaporated skim milk
2	cups low-fat Cheddar cheese (preferably very sharp)
1/3	cup instant nonfat dry milk
2	slices whole-wheat or multigrain bread, toasted, dried and blended into fine crumbs
2	tsp. melted butter

1. Put the onions in a skillet with enough water to cover. Cook until tender, stirring continuously. Drain in a colander.
2. Lightly coat a 9-inch pie plate with olive oil spray and arrange the onions evenly on the plate. Sprinkle with 1 teaspoon of the chicken seasoning and add the pepper to taste.
3. Pour the evaporated milk over the onions so as not to disturb the arrangement. Sprinkle evenly with the cheese. Combine the dry milk, bread crumbs and remaining 1 teaspoon chicken seasoning and sprinkle on the pie.
4. Bake at 350° for 25 to 30 minutes. Watch the crust; if it's browning too fast, cover the pie with aluminum foil.
5. Drizzle the top with the butter. Cool for a few minutes before cutting.

QUICHE LORRAINE

Nutrition Facts
Number of Servings: 4
Per Serving
- Calories: 425
- Saturated Fat: 7.297 grams
- Monounsaturated Fat: 4.565 grams
- Polyunsaturated Fat: 1.304 grams
- Total Fat: 15.48 grams
- Percentage of Calories From Fat: 34%

Crusty! Cheesy! Rich!

4	slices whole-wheat bread, toasted, dried and blended into crumbs
1/3	cup instant nonfat dry milk
	Freshly ground pepper
2	cups evaporated skim milk
4	large eggs
1	tbsp. minced fresh parsley
4	tsp. imitation bacon bits
1	chicken bouillon cube
1/4	tsp. onion powder
	Salt
1 1/4	cups shredded low-fat Swiss cheese (preferably aged)
1/4	tsp. garlic powder
4	tsp. melted butter

1. Spray the bottom and sides of a 9-inch pie plate with olive oil spray. Combine the bread crumbs, dry milk and pepper to taste, and with a few added drops of water, press into a pan and up the sides for a crust. Chill the crust for 30 minutes.
2. In a blender jar, starting with the evaporated milk, combine the evaporated milk, eggs, parsley, bacon bits, bouillon and onion powder. Blend, adding the salt to taste.
3. Pour slowly into the crust. Sprinkle evenly with the cheese and garlic powder. Bake at 350° for 35 minutes, or until the custard center is firm when a fork is inserted. Top evenly with the butter.

PIZZA

Nutrition Facts
Number of Servings: 6
Per Serving
- Calories: 371
- Saturated Fat: 6.599 grams
- Monounsaturated Fat: 6.174 grams
- Polyunsaturated Fat: 0.957 gram
- Total Fat: 14.98 grams
- Percentage of Calories From Fat: 35%

A satisfying rendering of the addictive pizza for those who crave that warm, cheesy wedge. (You can add low-fat turkey sausage to this pizza, but don't forget that it adds calories.)

6	slices whole-wheat or multigrain bread, toasted, dried and blended into medium-fine crumbs
2	cups instant nonfat dry milk
1–2	tbsp. dried oregano leaves
	Salt and freshly ground pepper
2	cups shredded low-fat mozzarella cheese
2	tbsp. minced fresh parsley
1	tbsp. minced fresh basil or $1/2$ tsp. dried basil
$3/4$	cup tomato sauce
$1/2$	tsp. garlic powder
$1\,1/4$	cups grated Parmesan cheese
4	tbsp. capers, well drained
	Strips of pimientos, drained (if desired but preferable)
2	tbsp. olive oil

1. Lightly coat a 12-inch pizza pan with olive oil spray.
2. In a bowl combine the bread crumbs, dry milk, oregano and salt and pepper to taste with enough water to moisten the mixture so that it can be patted out to line the pan and sides. Fill the crust with the mozzarella, parsley, basil and more of the pepper.
3. Carefully pour the tomato sauce over the filling. Sprinkle with the garlic powder and Parmesan. Decorate with the capers and pimientos if using. Sprinkle with more of the pepper if desired.
4. Bake at 400° for 20 to 25 minutes. If the crust is browning too rapidly, place a sheet of aluminium foil beneath the pan.
5. When the sides of the crust are browned, drizzle the pizza with the oil. Lift around the edges to prevent sticking, but leave in the pan to cool for a few minutes. Cut into 6 wedges.

A TIP FOR THE COOK

How does 1 gram of fat size up? A gram feels about as heavy as a paper clip, and it takes 454 grams to equal 1 pound. A 1-gram glob of fat would fill about 1/4 of a teaspoon. So a food with 8 grams of fat would have 2 teaspoons of it.

POTATO PANCAKES WITH APPLESAUCE

Nutrition Facts
Number of Servings: 1
Per Serving
- Calories: 473
- Saturated Fat: 6.631 grams
- Monounsaturated Fat: 4.212 grams
- Polyunsaturated Fat: 1.188 grams
- Total Fat: 15.3 grams
- Percentage of Calories From Fat: 28%

This will win your heart without adding to your waistline.

Pancakes:
1/3	cup finely shredded raw potatoes, drained
1/4	cup finely minced green onions or 2 tbsp. dry onion flakes
1	small egg, separated
1/3	cup instant nonfat dry milk
1	tsp. chicken seasoning
1	tsp. imitation bacon bits
	Pinch of ground nutmeg
	Pinch of freshly ground pepper
	Pinch of paprika
2	tsp. butter

Applesauce:
1	medium cooking apple, peeled, cored and sliced
1	tsp. sugar or honey
1	stick cinnamon, broken in half
1	whole clove

1. To make the pancakes: Press the potatoes and the fresh onions between paper towels to dry thoroughly.
2. In a bowl combine the potatoes, onions, egg yolk, dry milk, chicken seasoning, bacon bits, nutmeg, pepper and paprika.
3. Beat the egg white until stiff and extremely dry. Fold into the potato mixture.
4. Lightly coat a nonstick skillet with olive oil spray and heat over low heat. Spoon on 5 pancakes, flattening each with a spatula. Brown both sides very slowly, or the pancakes will have a raw taste.
5. Sprinkle with more of the paprika. Top with the butter.
6. To make the applesauce: Put all of the applesauce ingredients and $1/2$ cup water in a small skillet over medium heat and cover. Simmer until the apple slices are soft. Discard the spices.
7. Pour the apples and liquid into a blender jar. Blend until smooth.

A TIP FOR THE COOK

If you chop something smelly on your wooden chopping board (onions, fish, etc.), clean the board and rub lemon over it to remove the odor.

MUSHROOM SOUFFLÉ

Nutrition Facts
Number of Servings: 4
Per Serving
- Calories: 180
- Saturated Fat: 3.353 grams
- Monounsaturated Fat: 2.18 grams
- Polyunsaturated Fat: 0.599 gram
- Total Fat: 6.865 grams
- Percentage of Calories From Fat: 34%

This soufflé, studded with tidbits of mushrooms, gives the palate the illusion of meat—rich and aromatic. All in one bite.

2	cups sliced fresh mushrooms or ²/₃ cup sliced canned mushrooms
1	cup evaporated skim milk
1	slice white bread, torn into pieces
1	tbsp. cornstarch
1	oz. chopped onion
1	chicken bouillon cube
1	tbsp. minced fresh garlic or ¼ tsp. garlic powder
	Freshly ground pepper
2	large eggs, separated, plus 2 additional egg whites
¼	cup grated Parmesan cheese
	Ground nutmeg
2	tsp. melted butter

1. To cook the fresh mushrooms add 2 tablespoons water, 1/4 teaspoon salt and the mushrooms to a small nonstick saucepan. Place over high heat, cover and immediately reduce to low. Cook for about 6 minutes.
2. Drain the cooked or canned mushrooms and dry on paper towels. Chop very fine.
3. In a blender jar, starting with the milk, combine the milk, bread, cornstarch, onion, bouillon, garlic or garlic powder and pepper to taste. Blend until smooth, then pour into a large saucepan. Cook over medium heat, stirring, until thickened. Cool to lukewarm.
4. Gradually incorporate the egg yolks with a wooden spoon. Stir in the mushrooms.
5. Beat the 4 egg whites until stiff but not dry. Fold carefully into the mushroom mixture. Pour into a 4- to 6-cup ramekin or soufflé dish, lightly coated with olive oil spray. Sprinkle with the cheese and nutmeg.
6. Bake at 375° for 25 minutes, or until the center is firm. Drizzle with the butter.

CRAB AND CHEESE QUICHE

Nutrition Facts
  Number of Servings: 4
  Per Serving
  • Calories: 332
  • Saturated Fat: 5.893 grams
  • Monounsaturated Fat: 4.395 grams
  • Polyunsaturated Fat: 0.896 gram
  • Total Fat: 12.5 grams
  • Percentage of Calories From Fat: 35%

Salmon and crab are equally delicious in this "nouvelle cuisine" version of quiche.

  1   tsp. chicken seasoning
  1   medium (5 oz.) onion, thinly sliced into rings
  3   large eggs
  1/2 cup shredded low-fat Swiss cheese
  1   tbsp. grated Parmesan cheese
  2   cups evaporated skim milk
  1/4 tsp. garlic powder
     Salt and freshly ground pepper
  4   oz. crabmeat or canned salmon, drained and
     shredded
  1   tbsp. imitation bacon bits
     Ground nutmeg or mace
  2   tsp. melted butter

1. Add enough water to coat the bottom of a small non-stick skillet. Sprinkle with 1/2 teaspoon of the chicken seasoning and bring to a boil over medium-high heat. Add the onions and cook, stirring continuously, just until tender and lightly browned. Reserve.

2. In a blender jar combine the eggs, Swiss and Parmesan cheeses and 1 cup of the milk and blend until smooth. Pour into a mixing bowl and stir in the remaining 1 cup milk, the garlic powder and the remaining 1/2 tsp. chicken seasoning. Add the salt and pepper to taste. Fold in the crabmeat or salmon.

3. Pour into a 9-inch pie plate that has been lightly coated with olive oil spray. Sprinkle with the bacon bits. Arrange the onion on top. Sprinkle with the nutmeg or mace.

4. Bake at 400° for 10 minutes. Lower to 350° and bake for 25 to 30 minutes longer, or just until the custard center is firm when pressed. Drizzle with the butter.

"CANNELLONI" PIEDMONTESE

Nutrition Facts
  Number of Servings: 1
  Per Serving
  • Calories: 334
  • Saturated Fat: 4.358 grams
  • Monounsaturated Fat: 3.474 grams
  • Polyunsaturated Fat: 1.202 grams
  • Total Fat: 12.4 grams
  • Percentage of Calories From Fat: 31%

This rendition of cannelloni resembles a crepe stuffed with healthy fare and its traditional ricotta cheese.

1 ½ cups fresh spinach, washed, torn into small pieces
        and firmly packed
  ⅓ cup nonfat ricotta cheese
  ½ tsp. onion powder
  2 tsp. imitation bacon bits
  1 tsp. minced garlic
      Salt and freshly ground pepper
  1 slice multigrain bread, torn into pieces
  1 large egg
  ¼ cup evaporated skim milk
      Pinch of garlic powder
      Pinch of ground nutmeg
  1 tsp. melted butter

1. With the water clinging to the leaves, put the spinach in a small skillet, cover and steam over low heat until wilted. Squeeze out all of the moisture.
2. In a bowl combine the spinach, cheese, onion powder, bacon bits, garlic and salt and pepper to taste. As you blend the ingredients mash them with a fork. Reserve.
3. In a blender jar combine the bread, egg, milk, garlic powder and nutmeg and whirl until smooth, adding more of the salt and pepper to taste.
4. Coat a nonstick skillet with olive oil spray and pour the batter in, tilting the pan to spread evenly. Cook over medium heat, carefully checking the browning by lifting the edge of the pancake with a spatula. When it is brown flecked or evenly browned, turn. Do this carefully because the pancake will tear if turned too soon. Brown the other side.
5. Spread with the spinach-cheese filling and cover the skillet. Cook over the lowest possible heat until the cheese is melted. Fold in half or roll up and drizzle with the butter.

SOUFFLÉ DE CAROTTES

Nutrition Facts
  Number of Servings: 4
  Per Serving
  • Calories: 372
  • Saturated Fat: 5.986 grams
  • Monounsaturated Fat: 3.95 grams
  • Polyunsaturated Fat: 1.03 grams
  • Total Fat: 13.83 grams
  • Percentage of Calories From Fat: 33%

You will enjoy putting this together when all you have left in your refrigerator are carrots, cheese and eggs.

1	tbsp. cornstarch
1	cup evaporated skim milk
1	oz. chopped onion
1	chicken bouillon cube
1/8	tsp. ground nutmeg
1/8	tsp. dried thyme
8	small carrots, cooked
4	large eggs, separated
3/4	cup shredded low-fat sharp Cheddar cheese
1	tbsp. fresh minced parsley
	Freshly ground pepper
1/4	cup grated Parmesan cheese
2	tsp. melted butter

1. Dissolve the cornstarch in the milk and pour into a saucepan. Cook over medium heat, stirring, until thickened.
2. Pour the thickened cream into a blender jar. Add the onion, bouillon, nutmeg, thyme, carrots, egg yolks, Cheddar, parsley and pepper to taste and whirl until smooth.
3. Beat the egg whites until stiff but not dry. Fold carefully into the carrot mixture and pour into a 4- to 6-cup ramekin or soufflé dish. Sprinkle with the Parmesan.
4. Bake at 375° for about 30 minutes, or until the center is firm when pressed. Pour the melted butter evenly across the top.

STUFFED ZUCCHINI

Nutrition Facts
Number of Servings: 2
Per Serving
- Calories: 277
- Saturated Fat: 3.76 grams
- Monounsaturated Fat: 3.939 grams
- Polyunsaturated Fat: 0.701 gram
- Total Fat: 10.29 grams
- Percentage of Calories From Fat: 30%

A familiar sauce and taste, and what's more, it's satisfying.

2	medium (about 6 inches long) zucchini
	Salt
2/3	cup nonfat ricotta cheese or low-fat creamed cottage cheese
2	small cloves garlic, minced
2	tbsp. chopped fresh chives
2	tbsp. chopped fresh parsley
1	tsp. minced fresh oregano
1/4	tsp. crumbled dried basil
	Freshly ground pepper
2	oz. low-fat feta cheese or provolone cheese or Parmesan cheese, grated
1/2	cup low-sodium tomato sauce or puree
2	tsp. olive oil

1. Cut the unpeeled zucchini in half lengthwise and hollow it out. Sprinkle with the salt and dry on paper towels.
2. In a small bowl combine the ricotta and seasonings, reserving some of the garlic and oregano and adding the pepper to taste. Stuff each zucchini half.
3. Arrange in an ovenproof dish. Sprinkle with the feta, provolone or Parmesan and pour the tomato sauce or puree over the top. Sprinkle with the reserved garlic and oregano.
4. Add 1 inch water, cover with aluminum foil and bake at 350° for about 30 minutes, or until the zucchini is tender. Uncover, increase the oven temperature to 450° and bake until browned. Drizzle with the oil.

Eggs,
Cheeses
and
Vegetables
❖

EGGPLANT PARMIGIANA

Nutrition Facts
Number of Servings: 2
Per Serving
- Calories: 120
- Saturated Fat: 1.936 grams
- Monounsaturated Fat: 2.399 grams
- Polyunsaturated Fat: 0.293 gram
- Total Fat: 4.875 grams
- Percentage of Calories From Fat: 35%

If seeing is believing, eating is convincing. No one could tell this one apart from the "real thing."

4	¾-inch-thick slices unpeeled eggplant
	Salt and freshly ground pepper
2	tbsp. grated low-fat mozzarella cheese
2	tbsp. grated Parmesan cheese
⅓	cup nonfat ricotta cheese or low-fat creamed cottage cheese
⅓	cup low-sodium tomato sauce
2	tbsp. buttermilk or yogurt
1	tbsp. minced fresh parsley
¼	tsp. crumbled oregano
1	clove garlic, minced
1	tsp. olive oil

1. Put 1 inch water in a large skillet and add the eggplant. Simmer, uncovered and turning, until barely tender. Pat dry with paper towels and let it drain.
2. Arrange the slices in a baking dish, side by side. Sprinkle with the salt and pepper to taste and cover evenly with the mozzarella and Parmesan.
3. In a bowl combine the ricotta or cottage cheese, tomato sauce, buttermilk or yogurt, parsley, oregano and garlic. Spread over the eggplant.
4. Bake at 350° for 25 minutes, or until the eggplant is soft and the top is browned. Drizzle with the oil.

RATATOUILLE NIÇOISE

Nutrition Facts

Number of Servings: 4

Per Serving

- Calories: 96
- Saturated Fat: 0.52 gram
- Monounsaturated Fat: 2.523 grams
- Polyunsaturated Fat: 0.454 gram
- Total Fat: 3.892 grams
- Percentage of Calories From Fat: 33%

In France ratatouille is cooked very slowly so that each vegetable infuses the others with its aroma and taste. The dish tastes better when it has been sitting for a time or overnight to bind the flavors further.

2	cups diced peeled eggplant
4	medium cloves garlic, minced
1	tbsp. minced fresh basil or ¼ tsp. crumbled dried basil
1	green pepper, cut into strips
1	red bell pepper, cut into strips
2	cups diced unpeeled zucchini
½	cup low-sodium tomato sauce or puree
	Salt and freshly ground pepper
2	medium unpeeled tomatoes, diced
1	tbsp. virgin olive oil

1. Simmer the eggplant in 2 tablespoons water in a large skillet, adding the garlic and basil. When almost tender, add the green and red peppers and cook until tender. Then add the zucchini, tomato sauce or puree and salt and ground pepper to taste.
2. Cover and reduce to very low heat. Simmer for 15 minutes, then add the diced tomatoes. Cover and continue simmering slowly until the liquid is absorbed. Add more of the salt, if necessary.
3. Sprinkle with the oil and toss lightly. Let it set for several hours or overnight. It is best served at room temperature.

Eggs,
Cheeses
and
Vegetables
❖

GINGER-GLAZED CARROTS

Nutrition Facts
  Number of Servings: 4
  Per Serving
  • Calories: 103
  • Saturated Fat: 0.513 gram
  • Monounsaturated Fat: 1.362 grams
  • Polyunsaturated Fat: 1.519 grams
  • Total Fat: 3.635 grams
  • Percentage of Calories From Fat: 30%

Sweet and sour, this Chinese-inspired side dish not only is low in calories but also singles out the healthful effects of carrots. Tastes like a dessert.

1   lb. carrots
3   tsp. honey
1   tsp. grated fresh ginger or ¼ tsp. ground ginger
3   tbsp. low-sodium soy sauce
1   clove garlic, minced, or ¼ tsp. garlic powder
1   tbsp. sesame oil

1. Cut the carrots into strips the size of slender french fries. In a skillet combine the carrots, honey and ginger with enough water to cover. Simmer, covered, over medium heat until the carrots are barely tender.
2. Increase the heat and cook, uncovered, until the liquid has evaporated. Then quick-stir the carrots to give them a caramel color.
3. Add the soy sauce, garlic or garlic powder and oil. Toss and serve warm.

BROCCOLI AU GRATIN

Nutrition Facts
Number of Servings: 2
Per Serving
- Calories: 295
- Saturated Fat: 1.639 grams
- Monounsaturated Fat: 4.453 grams
- Polyunsaturated Fat: 0.927 gram
- Total Fat: 9.842 grams
- Percentage of Calories From Fat: 30%

The benefits of broccoli are no longer a secret. But preparing this miracle food still is. Here is one version that makes it a favorite vegetable.

⅓	cup low-fat ricotta cheese or low-fat creamed cottage cheese
1	large egg
1½	tbsp. lemon juice
1	cup evaporated skim milk
1	tbsp. fresh minced parsley
2	cloves garlic, minced
	Pinch of ground nutmeg or mace
	Salt and freshly ground pepper
1	cup cooked broccoli spears, cut into 2-inch pieces
2	tsp. imitation bacon bits
1	slice whole-wheat bread, toasted, dried and blended into fine crumbs
2	tsp. olive oil

1. In a blender jar combine the cheese, egg, lemon juice, milk, parsley, garlic and nutmeg or mace. Blend until smooth. Add the salt and pepper to taste.
2. Arrange the broccoli in a 3- to 4-cup ramekin or baking dish and cover with the cheese mixture. Sprinkle with the bacon bits and bake at 350° for 30 to 35 minutes, or until the custard is nearly set.
3. Increase the temperature to 400°. Sprinkle the bread crumbs over the top and bake until lightly browned. Drizzle with the oil.

Eggs,
Cheeses
and
Vegetables
❖

SPINACH PIE

Nutrition Facts
  Number of Servings: 2
  Per Serving
  • Calories: 334
  • Saturated Fat: 4.785 grams
  • Monounsaturated Fat: 4.394 grams
  • Polyunsaturated Fat: 0.753 gram
  • Total Fat: 11.14 grams
  • Percentage of Calories From Fat: 28%

Feta cheese is a staple of Greek cooking. It adds a bit of the *je ne sais quoi* of sharp country fare to anything—even to spinach!

1	10-oz. package frozen chopped spinach
1	envelope dry onion soup mix or 1 tsp. onion powder
2/3	cup chopped green onions
1/2	cup fat-free egg substitute
2	oz. finely crumbled feta cheese
1/2	cup evaporated skim milk
2	oz. natural brown rice wafers, thin Norwegian flat bread or any super-flat dried bread
	Salt and freshly ground pepper
	Ground nutmeg
	Cinnamon
2	tsp. olive oil

1. Cook the spinach according to package directions and drain thoroughly. Squeeze dry. Reserve in a mixing bowl.
2. In a skillet mix a small amount of water and the soup mix or onion powder and quickly cook until the onions are tender. Drain and mix well with the reserved spinach. Stir in the egg substitute and cheese. Add the milk and stir to mix well.
3. Preheat the oven to 350°. Thinly coat a medium-size baking dish with olive oil spray. Arrange a third of the spinach mixture at the bottom of the dish. Make another layer using a third of the wafers or bread. Sprinkle with the salt and pepper.
4. Repeat these layers until the spinach mixture and wafers or bread are used up, ending with the wafers or bread. Sprinkle the last layer with a touch of the nutmeg and cinnamon. Lightly sprinkle the top with water to dampen.
5. Bake for about 20 to 25 minutes, or until browned and slightly puffed. Pour the oil evenly across the top. Serve warm.

BAKED MACARONI AND CHEESE

Nutrition Facts
  Number of Servings: 4
  Per Serving
  • Calories: 428
  • Saturated Fat: 7.622 grams
  • Monounsaturated Fat: 5.238 grams
  • Polyunsaturated Fat: 1.089 grams
  • Total Fat: 15.9 grams
  • Percentage of Calories From Fat: 33%

This macaroni bake has two cheeses, milk, eggs—even butter. Do you dare prepare this?

1 1/4 cups uncooked elbow macaroni
   2   cups evaporated skim milk
   4   eggs
   1   cup shredded low-fat Swiss cheese
   1   clove garlic, minced, or 1/4 tsp. garlic powder
       Salt and freshly ground pepper
  1/4 cup grated Parmesan cheese or Romano cheese
       Ground nutmeg
   4   tsp. melted butter

1. Cook the macaroni in boiling salted water. This will render 2 1/4 cups cooked pasta. Drain.
2. Arrange the macaroni in a small baking dish.
3. In a blender jar combine the milk, eggs, Swiss cheese and garlic or garlic powder and whirl until smooth. Add the salt and pepper to taste.
4. Pour over the macaroni. Top with the Parmesan or Romano and sprinkle lightly with the nutmeg.
5. Bake at 350° for 30 to 35 minutes, or until the center feels nearly firm when touched. Watch it and cover if necessary. Pour the melted butter evenly on top.

STUFFED ACORN SQUASH

Nutrition Facts
  Number of Servings: 4
  Per Serving
  • Calories: 260
  • Saturated Fat: 0.94 gram
  • Monounsaturated Fat: 1.128 grams
  • Polyunsaturated Fat: 0.625 gram
  • Total Fat: 4.673 grams
  • Percentage of Calories From Fat: 16%

A sweet treat to go with your lean turkey at Thanksgiving.

1	large acorn squash, halved and seeded
2	large eggs
1	tsp. vanilla
2	tbsp. brown sugar
1/2	tsp. pumpkin pie spice
2/3	cup low-fat ricotta cheese or low-fat creamed cottage cheese
1	tsp. onion powder
2	slices white bread, toasted, dried and blended into crumbs
	Salt

1. In a 9-inch baking pan place the squash upside down and add 2 tablespoons water. Cover with aluminum foil and bake at 350° for about 40 minutes, or until the pulp is tender. Scoop out all of the meat, but keep the shells.
2. In a blender jar combine the eggs, vanilla, squash meat, sugar, spice, cheese, onion powder and two-thirds of the bread crumbs. Whirl until smooth, adding water if necessary. Salt to taste.
3. Spoon the mixture into the shells. Sprinkle with the remaining bread crumbs. Bake at 450°, uncovered, for about 10 minutes, or until puffed and firm.

Eggs,
Cheeses
and
Vegetables
❖

OMELETTE MOUSSELINE

Nutrition Facts
Number of Servings: 2
Per Serving
- Calories: 94
- Saturated Fat: 0.783 gram
- Monounsaturated Fat: 0.96 gram
- Polyunsaturated Fat: 0.357 gram
- Total Fat: 2.552 grams
- Percentage of Calories From Fat: 25%

This omelette is as light as a feather. Don't overcook.

1	large egg, separated, plus 3 additional egg whites
1	tsp. chicken seasoning
1/4	tsp. minced fresh chervil
1	tbsp. minced fresh chives
1/2	tsp. minced fresh dill or pinch of dried dill
1	tbsp. minced fresh oregano or 1/4 tsp. dried oregano
1/2	tsp. minced fresh parsley
1/2	tbsp. minced fresh garlic or 1/8 tsp. garlic powder Freshly ground pepper
1	oz. grated fat-free Cheddar cheese

1. In a bowl combine the egg yolk with the chicken seasoning, herbs, garlic or garlic powder and pepper to taste. Beat with a whisk until light in color. Beat the 4 egg whites until soft peaks form. Quickly beat the yolk/herb mixture into the egg whites.
2. Preheat a large nonstick skillet over medium heat and pour in the egg mixture, tilting the pan for even distribution. Cover the pan for a few minutes.
3. With a spatula lift the edge to check the underside of the omelette. Sprinkle the center with the cheese. Cook for an extra few minutes. The center of the omelette should be *baveuse*, or moist.
4. Carefully flip one side over the other. Cook for 1 to 2 minutes longer. Serve at once.

SEAFOOD

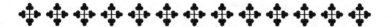

The merits of seafood hardly need to be emphasized. We are told that we should eat four to five portions of fish per week. To me, fish used to mean going to a restaurant and ordering an elegant salmon steak or broiled shrimp stuffed with crab—nothing like the smelly pieces of fish lying on ice in my local supermarket.

Eating fish in a restaurant five times a week became ruinous to our pocketbook. I needed to learn how to create these chic, saucy seafood preparations right at home. And I did.

In the following recipes you will find our plantation calderata, oysters au gratin, fillet of sole Normandy (with two sauces and rolled around shrimp) and other specialties that will have you rushing to the nearest fish market.

These are only samples of the endless ways you can serve seafood and entertain your health-conscious friends. These dishes are a showcase of culinary masterpieces. Why not create your own?

If the mood strikes you and you want that old "fish fry" taste, here is my quick and easy method: Mix 1/3 cup of dry milk powder with 1 teaspoon of onion powder. Dip fresh fillets of sole or flounder in this mixture, coating both sides. Lightly coat a nonstick skillet with olive oil spray and heat it. Cook the fillets slowly on both sides just until the fish is done and browned.

You can also make my quick tartar sauce: Mix 1 tablespoon of plain yogurt, 1/4 cup of chopped fresh chives, 1 tablespoon of imitation mayonnaise, 1/4 teaspoon each of salt and pepper, 1 teaspoon of chopped capers and lots of fresh lime juice. Put this sauce over the fish and cover with the lid for a minute or two.

SHRIMP CREOLE

Nutrition Facts
  Number of Servings: 1
  Per Serving
  • Calories: 440
  • Saturated Fat: 1.466 grams
  • Monounsaturated Fat: 3.974 grams
  • Polyunsaturated Fat: 2.18 grams
  • Total Fat: 9.267 grams
  • Percentage of Calories From Fat: 18%

This evokes jazz nights and hot spices. Served with plain brown rice, this dish takes on gargantuan portions yet has a lilliputian calorie and fat count.

¼	cup minced onions
2	stalks celery, chopped
½	cup tomato sauce or puree
½	green pepper, chopped
½	cup sliced fresh mushrooms or ¼ cup sliced canned mushrooms
1	crumbled dried bay leaf
¼	tsp. crumbled dried tarragon
1	tbsp. minced fresh parsley
1 ½	tsp. fresh dill or ½ tsp. dried dill
⅛	tsp. cayenne pepper or hot pepper sauce
½	cup clam juice
8	oz. uncooked shrimp, peeled and deveined
	Juice of 1 lime
	Salt
1	tsp. olive oil
	Cooked brown rice (if desired)

1. In a saucepan combine the onions, celery and tomato sauce or puree. Cover and simmer for 5 minutes.
2. Add the green peppers, fresh mushrooms (the canned ones are added later), bay leaf, tarragon, parsley, dill, cayenne pepper or hot pepper sauce and clam juice. Cover and simmer for about 15 minutes, or until the mushrooms are tender.
3. Add the shrimp and canned mushrooms if using. Cover and simmer for about 5 minutes, or until the shrimp are tender. Don't overcook the shrimp.
4. Add the lime juice and the salt to taste. Drizzle the oil atop evenly. Serve over the rice if using.

A TIP FOR THE COOK

To determine the percentage of fat in a food or recipe, multiply the grams of fat by 9 to get the number of calories from fat. (Each gram of fat contains 9 calories.) Then divide by the total number of calories.

COD CROQUETTES

Nutrition Facts
Number of Servings: 2
Per Serving
- Calories: 326
- Saturated Fat: 1.608 grams
- Monounsaturated Fat: 2.078 grams
- Polyunsaturated Fat: 4.622 grams
- Total Fat: 9.652 grams
- Percentage of Calories From Fat: 26%

Any leftover fish will do for this recipe.

2	cups flaked cooked cod or other fish
2	slices whole-wheat or multigrain bread, toasted, dried and blended into fine crumbs
1	cup minced cooked mushrooms or 1 cup minced canned mushrooms, drained
2	tbsp. minced fresh parsley
2	tbsp. minced fresh chives
4	medium cloves garlic, minced
2	tbsp. imitation mayonnaise
	Salt and freshly ground pepper
1/3	cup instant nonfat dry milk or dry soy milk
1	tsp. onion powder
	Lime or lemon wedges for garnish

1. In a mixing bowl finely crumble the cooked fish with a fork and add the bread crumbs, mushrooms, parsley, chives, garlic, mayonnaise and salt and pepper to taste. Mix thoroughly, adding water if necessary, and form into 4 patties.
2. Mix the dry milk or soy milk with the onion powder. Roll the patties in this mixture.
3. Lightly coat a nonstick skillet with olive oil spray and brown the patties slowly over medium to low heat, turning often. These patties will be crusty on the outside and moist on the inside.
4. Make your own tartar sauce (see the directions on page 87) or any low-fat sauce of your choice. Serve surrounded with lots of the lime or lemon wedges.

CALDERATA

Nutrition Facts
  Number of Servings: 1
  Per Serving
  • Calories: 436
  • Saturated Fat: 1.623 grams
  • Monounsaturated Fat: 6.936 grams
  • Polyunsaturated Fat: 1.653 grams
  • Total Fat: 11.44 grams
  • Percentage of Calories From Fat: 23%

Served by Portuguese fishermen after their day's catch, here is the version that became our plantation's customary fare, since we "grew" telapia fish in our ponds.

2   medium tomatoes, very thinly sliced
1   small (3–4 oz.) potato, very thinly sliced
6   oz. fillet of cod, cut into chunks
1   medium (5 oz.) onion, very thinly sliced
4   cloves garlic, minced
     Salt and freshly ground pepper
     Crushed red, cayenne or minced jalapeño pepper
     or hot pepper sauce
¼   cup tomato sauce or puree
2   tsp. olive oil

1. In a medium baking dish make a layer of half of the tomato slices, then half of the potatoes, half of the fish and half of the onions, seasoning as you go with the garlic, salt, ground pepper and hot pepper. Repeat the layers and the seasonings. Pour on the tomato sauce or puree.
2. Cover and bake at 350° for about 30 to 35 minutes, watching it closely. Most of the liquid should be evaporated, but it should not be allowed to dry.
3. Drizzle with the oil and serve warm.

FILLET OF SOLE NORMANDY

Nutrition Facts
Number of Servings: 2
Per Serving
- Calories: 377
- Saturated Fat: 4.428 grams
- Monounsaturated Fat: 2.279 grams
- Polyunsaturated Fat: 1.414 grams
- Total Fat: 9.673 grams
- Percentage of Calories From Fat: 23%

A simple fillet becomes the centerpiece of an elegant dinner party.

8 oz. fillet of sole
8 oz. medium uncooked shrimp, peeled and deveined
1 cup sliced fresh mushrooms or ½ cup whole canned button mushrooms
Salt and freshly ground pepper
Juice of 1 lime
Bouquet garni of 1 dried bay leaf, 3 whole black peppercorns and ¼ tsp. dried tarragon, tied in cheesecloth or placed in a metal tea ball
1 tbsp. cornstarch
½ cup evaporated skim milk
1 tsp. chicken seasoning
¼ tsp. onion powder
Pinch of ground nutmeg
1 tbsp. tomato sauce and 1 tbsp. butter, mixed and warmed
1 lime, cut into thin wedges

1. Cut the fish into pieces large enough to wrap around each shrimp. Tightly roll each piece of fillet around a shrimp and secure with a toothpick.
2. In a medium skillet simmer the fresh mushrooms with 1 tablespoon water, 1/8 teaspoon of the salt and a dash of the pepper just until soft, about 5 minutes. (If using the canned mushrooms, just warm them up.) Cover and keep warm.
3. Arrange the fish rolls in a larger skillet with 1/2 inch water, 1 tablespoon of the lime juice and the bouquet garni and bring to a boil. Reduce the heat to low and barely simmering, poach the fish, turning it, for about 10 minutes, or just until the fish is no longer translucent inside. Remove the bouquet garni.
4. In a smaller skillet dissolve the cornstarch in the cold milk, then add the chicken seasoning and onion powder. Cook over medium heat, stirring constantly, until thickened. Mix in the remaining lime juice, nutmeg and more of the salt and pepper to taste. With a spatula move the fillet rolls onto a serving platter. Pour the fish liquid and the sauce evenly over the rolls.
5. Drain the mushrooms, pat dry and arrange around the edge of the platter. Dot the rolls with the warmed tomato-butter sauce. Take an extra dish with thin wedges of lime to the table.

BAKED STUFFED FISH

Nutrition Facts
  Number of Servings: 1
  Per Serving
  • Calories: 777
  • Saturated Fat: 7.141 grams
  • Monounsaturated Fat: 11.7 grams
  • Polyunsaturated Fat: 5.286 grams
  • Total Fat: 30.51 grams
  • Percentage of Calories From Fat: 35%

At Cape Sounion in Greece we tasted the local fish prepared in this fashion. I have used small bluefish and trout, but lake bass and even cod and perch will do justice to this healthy dish. In Taxco I used a small, black fish whose name I cannot even pronounce, and it was delicious.

1	whole fish (about 1 1/4 lbs.), cleaned and head and tail removed, if preferred (I like to leave the head on because it makes a wonderful gelatin while it cooks.)
1/4	tsp. ground thyme
	Salt and freshly ground pepper
1	stalk celery, finely chopped
1/2	cup thinly sliced carrots
2	oz. onion, sliced into thin rings
1	unpeeled lime, sliced into thin rings
2–3	(or more) cloves garlic, minced
1	tbsp. crumbled oregano
2	dried bay leaves
2	tsp. olive oil
	Lemon wedges

1. Preheat the oven to 350°.
2. Wash the inside of the fish and dry with plenty of paper towels. Dust with the thyme, salt and pepper.
3. In a bowl combine the celery, carrots, onions, lime, garlic and oregano. Stuff the fish with half of the mixture and arrange in a baking dish. Add 1 inch water and the bay leaves.
4. Cover the fish with the remaining celery mixture. Sprinkle with more of the salt and pepper. Cover the dish with aluminum foil and bake for about 20 to 25 minutes, or until the fish is no longer translucent inside. Remove the bay leaves.
5. Uncover and drizzle the oil over the fish. Leave in the oven, uncovered, for 1 to 2 minutes. Serve hot, with lots of lemon wedges on the side.

A Tip for the Cook

To get more juice from a lemon, roll the lemon on a work surface before cutting and squeezing.

SCALLOPS ST. JACQUES

Nutrition Facts
  Number of Servings: 2
  Per Serving
  • Calories: 291
  • Saturated Fat: 2.761 grams
  • Monounsaturated Fat: 1.474 grams
  • Polyunsaturated Fat: 0.712 gram
  • Total Fat: 5.772 grams
  • Percentage of Calories From Fat: 18%

Served in the traditional white *coquilles* (shells), this dish is exceptionally refined as well as tasty. Quick and easy to make.

1   tbsp. white vinegar
1   dried bay leaf
1   tsp. pickling spice
1/4   tsp. crumbled dried tarragon
8   oz. raw scallops, halved
1/4   cup grated Parmesan cheese
2   large cloves garlic, pureed
1/2   cup nonfat yogurt
     Freshly ground pepper
2   slices white bread, toasted, dried and blended into
     fine crumbs
     Juice of 1/2 lemon
1   lime or lemon, cut into wedges

1. In a skillet combine 1 cup water and the vinegar, bay leaf, spice and tarragon. Bring to a rolling boil. Immediately lower the heat and add the scallops.
2. Simmer for about 2 minutes, or until the scallops are no longer translucent inside. Remove the scallops, drain and arrange in 4 baking shells or 2 au gratin ramekins or baking dishes.
3. Combine the cheese, garlic, yogurt and pepper to taste. Pour over the scallops. Top with the bread crumbs and the lemon juice.
5. Broil for 5 minutes, or until hot throughout and slightly browned. Serve with the lime or lemon wedges.

QUICK CURRIED SHRIMP

Nutrition Facts
Number of Servings: 1
Per Serving
- Calories: 320
- Saturated Fat: 5.35 grams
- Monounsaturated Fat: 2.534 grams
- Polyunsaturated Fat: 0.798 gram
- Total Fat: 9.418 grams
- Percentage of Calories From Fat: 26%

So fast that you will think it came cooked in a package!
On top of cooked brown or white rice, this dish is more
than satisfying.

2	tsp. cornstarch
1/2	cup evaporated skim milk
1	tsp. chicken seasoning
1/2	tsp. curry powder (preferably Madras type)
1/8	tsp. ground cardamom
1/8	tsp. garlic powder
	Pinch of freshly ground pepper
	Pinch of ground nutmeg
	Pinch of crushed red pepper
4	oz. cooked shrimp, peeled and deveined
2	tsp. melted butter

1. In a saucepan dissolve the cornstarch in the cold milk.
   Add the remaining ingredients except the shrimp and
   butter.
2. Cook over medium heat, stirring constantly, until
   thickened. Add the shrimp and warm until heated
   through.
3. Top with the melted butter.

OYSTERS AU GRATIN

Nutrition Facts
Number of Servings: 2
Per Serving
- Calories: 357
- Saturated Fat: 4.438 grams
- Monounsaturated Fat: 2.109 grams
- Polyunsaturated Fat: 1.154 grams
- Total Fat: 8.579 grams
- Percentage of Calories From Fat: 22%

Is it true what they say about oysters? In any case they seem to be one of men's favorite foods. If you bake these in white shells or individual au gratin dishes, you will be authentic.

1	cup evaporated skim milk
2	cloves garlic, minced or pureed
2	tbsp. cornstarch
1	tsp. chicken seasoning
1/4	tsp. onion powder
2	tbsp. lime or lemon juice
1/2	tsp. brandy flavoring (if desired)
1	cup cooked or canned sliced mushrooms, drained
8	oz. oysters, drained
	Salt and freshly ground pepper
	Ground nutmeg
1	tbsp. grated Parmesan cheese
1	slice white bread, toasted, dried and blended into crumbs
1/4	tsp. crumbled dried tarragon
1	tbsp. melted butter

1. In a medium saucepan combine the milk and garlic. Add the cornstarch and stir to dissolve. Add the chicken seasoning and onion powder.
2. Cook over medium heat, stirring constantly, until thickened. Stir in the lime or lemon juice, flavoring if using, mushrooms and oysters. Mix thoroughly.
3. Add the salt and pepper to taste and 1/4 teaspoon of the nutmeg. Spoon the mixture into shells or au gratin baking dishes.
4. Mix the Parmesan, bread crumbs, tarragon and a dash more of the salt, pepper and nutmeg. Sprinkle over the oyster mixture. Bake at 350° for 15 minutes, or until the top is browned and the mixture is bubbly. Drizzle evenly with the melted butter.

A TIP FOR THE COOK

Oyster lovers, take care. Oysters can contain the *Vibrio vulnificus* bacteria, which can cause serious illness and even death in some people. To be sure you kill the bacteria, follow these cooking guidelines:

• Oysters in the shell should be boiled for 3 to 5 minutes after the shells open or steamed for 4 to 9 minutes.

• Shucked oysters can be boiled or simmered for at least 3 minutes or until the edges curl, fried in oil for at least 3 minutes, broiled 3 inches from the heat for 3 minutes or baked at 450° for 10 minutes.

SHRIMP STUFFED WITH CRAB

Nutrition Facts
  Number of Servings: 2
  Per Serving
  • Calories: 372
  • Saturated Fat: 1.905 grams
  • Monounsaturated Fat: 2.09 grams
  • Polyunsaturated Fat: 5.282 grams
  • Total Fat: 10.5 grams
  • Percentage of Calories From Fat: 25%

This elegant inducement will captivate the most
jaded gourmet.

12	oz. uncooked jumbo shrimp, unpeeled
1	tbsp. cornstarch
1/2	cup evaporated skim milk
1/8	tsp. crumbled dried tarragon
1/8	tsp. garlic powder
4	oz. crabmeat, drained (save 1 tbsp. of the liquid)
	Juice of 1 lime or lemon
	Salt and freshly ground pepper
	Pinch of ground nutmeg
	Pinch of paprika
2	tbsp. imitation mayonnaise

1. Peel and devein the shrimp, leaving the tails on. Partially
   cut into each shrimp lengthwise down the back (where
   deveined), making a cavity for the stuffing.
2. In a small skillet dissolve the cornstarch in the milk.
   Add the tarragon and garlic powder. Cook over medium heat, stirring constantly, until thickened.
3. Remove and add the crab and lime or lemon juice.
   Mix well, adding the salt and pepper to taste. Fill the
   shrimp, patting the mixture firmly into the cavity.
4. Arrange the shrimp side by side in a small baking dish.
   Dust with the nutmeg and paprika. Add 1 tablespoon
   water and the crabmeat liquid to the pan. Bake,
   uncovered, at 350° for 20 to 30 minutes.
5. Melt mayonnaise over each shrimp and serve warm.

SHRIMP TERIYAKI

Nutrition Facts
Number of Servings: 2
Per Serving
- Calories: 597
- Saturated Fat: 1.523 grams
- Monounsaturated Fat: 3.422 grams
- Polyunsaturated Fat: 2.951 grams
- Total Fat: 8.805 grams
- Percentage of Calories From Fat: 13%

Only a small portion of your daily calorie quota. Low in fat! Treat yourself to another dish of your choice to complement. Or eat the whole thing.

8	oz. uncooked large shrimp, unpeeled
2	cloves garlic, minced
1/4	cup low-sodium soy sauce
1/4	tsp. prepared mustard
1	tbsp. tomato sauce
1	drop hot pepper sauce
1	tbsp. sugar
1	tsp. wine vinegar
1	tbsp. minced fresh ginger or 1/4 tsp. (or more) ground ginger
1	tbsp. peanut oil (or other if not available)

1. Peel and devein the shrimp, leaving the tails on.
2. In a saucepan combine the remaining ingredients except the oil and boil for 1 minute. Pour into a bowl and add the shrimp. Cover and marinate in the refrigerator for at least 3 hours, turning often.
3. Arrange the shrimp on skewers. If wooden skewers are used, soak them in water first to prevent burning. Broil for approximately 5 minutes on each side, basting often with the oil.

SOLE WITH GRAPE SAUCE

Nutrition Facts
  Number of Servings: 2
  Per Serving
  • Calories: 297
  • Saturated Fat: 4.13 grams
  • Monounsaturated Fat: 2.016 grams
  • Polyunsaturated Fat: 0.743 gram
  • Total Fat: 7.742 grams
  • Percentage of Calories From Fat: 23%

No doubt Bacchus trampled his feet to crush these sweet grapes, which, when blended with the tartness of spinach, create a symbolic delight. Quick and easy, too.

8	oz. fillet of sole
1/2	cup cooked spinach, drained and chopped
3/4	cup chopped green onions
1	tbsp. chopped fresh parsley
1 1/2	tsp. fresh minced dill or 1/2 tsp. dried dill
1/2	tsp. crumbled oregano
	Salt and freshly ground pepper
1	tbsp. cornstarch
1/2	cup evaporated skim milk
	Dash of ground nutmeg
1	cup firm sweet seedless green grapes
	Juice of 1 lime
1	tbsp. melted butter

1. Rinse the fillet and pat dry with plenty of paper towels. Cut into 4 equal portions. Squeeze the spinach dry.
2. In a small amount of water boil the onions for 1 minute. Drain well.
3. In a bowl combine the spinach, onions, parsley, dill, oregano and salt and pepper to taste. Spread the filling on each fish fillet. Roll the fillets and secure with toothpicks. Arrange, close to each other, in a small baking dish.
4. In a small skillet dissolve the cornstarch in the cold milk. Add the nutmeg and cook over medium heat, stirring, until thickened. Reserve.
5. Coarsely chop the grapes and put them and their juices into a small skillet. Add as little water as possible to prevent burning as you simmer the grapes for 5 minutes, or until soft and all of the liquid has evaporated.
6. Stir the grapes into the white sauce and pour over the fish. Bake, covered, at 350° for 15 to 20 minutes, or until the fish is no longer translucent inside.
7. Add the lime juice to taste to the pan liquid. Pour the butter on the fillet. Cover with enough of the pan liquid to make a glaze.

SPINACH RING WITH SALMON

Nutrition Facts
  Number of Servings: 2
  Per Serving
  • Calories: 446
  • Saturated Fat: 3.976 grams
  • Monounsaturated Fat: 5.281 grams
  • Polyunsaturated Fat: 6.451 grams
  • Total Fat: 17.92 grams
  • Percentage of Calories From Fat: 35%

Looks great. Tastes luscious. Have your salmon and spinach—and eat them, too!

1	10-oz. package frozen chopped spinach
2	slices whole-wheat bread, torn into pieces
1	tsp. chicken seasoning
1	tsp. onion powder
	Dash of ground nutmeg
1	cup evaporated skim milk
1/2	tsp. brandy flavoring (if desired)
2	large eggs, beaten
1	cup sliced fresh mushrooms or 1/3 cup sliced canned mushrooms
	Salt
4	oz. canned salmon, drained and flaked (remove all bony cartilage)
2	tbsp. imitation mayonnaise
2	tsp. lime juice
	Freshly ground pepper

1. Cook the spinach according to the package directions; drain and squeeze dry. Reserve.
2. In a blender jar combine the bread, chicken seasoning, onion powder, nutmeg and milk. Whirl until smooth. Pour the mixture into a small saucepan and cook over medium heat, stirring, until thickened. Remove from the stove.
3. Add the brandy flavoring if using, spinach and eggs. Mix well. Pour the mixture into a 3-cup ring mold. Set the mold in a baking pan and add 1 inch hot water to the pan. Bake at 350° for 30 minutes, or until the center is firm when pressed and the liquid has evaporated.
4. Cook the fresh mushrooms with $1/8$ teaspoon of the salt and 1 tablespoon water, covered, until soft. If using the canned mushrooms, only reheat in their own liquid.
5. Drain the mushrooms. Add the salmon, mayonnaise, lime juice, pepper to taste and more of the salt to taste and mix. Heat slowly over low heat until warm.
6. Unmold the hot spinach ring onto a serving plate and fill the center with the warm salmon mixture. If you prefer this dish cold, refrigerate the spinach mold and don't warm the salmon mixture.

CURRIED TUNABURGERS

Nutrition Facts
Number of Servings: 2
Per Serving
- Calories: 116
- Saturated Fat: 0.426 gram
- Monounsaturated Fat: 0.476 gram
- Polyunsaturated Fat: 0.677 gram
- Total Fat: 2.136 grams
- Percentage of Calories From Fat: 16%

When "hamburger obsession" strikes, have this tunaburger on whole-wheat toast, topped with mustard and a slice each of tomato and cucumber. Guaranteed to break the high-fat, high-calorie momentum.

1   slice whole-wheat bread, toasted, dried and blended into medium-fine crumbs
4   oz. tuna, well drained
1   tbsp. minced onions
1/2   tsp. curry powder (or 1 tsp. Maggi seasoning, if preferred)
1/4   tsp. dill
1/4   tsp. garlic powder
1/4   tsp. ground cumin
     Salt and freshly ground pepper
1/4   tsp. prepared mustard
1   tbsp. minced fresh parsley
     Skim milk

1. In a bowl combine all of the ingredients, using enough of the milk to moisten the mixture so that it can be shaped into 2 thin, firm patties, and adding the salt and pepper to taste.
2. Broil for about 6 minutes on each side, or until browned and crisp. If you prefer, you can cook the patties in a nonstick skillet, turning often, until browned on the outside.

CHICKEN

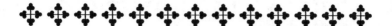

Chicken has been praised since medieval times. The Persians cooked their birds in pomegranate juice or concentrated pomegranate sauce. At times chicken was perfumed with cardamom pods and lemon juice. The French simmer their *poulet* in wine and cream (evaporated skim milk for calorie and fat counters!).

In Casablanca our family was treated to chicken with prunes over couscous. In Suriname we sampled tender morsels of chicken basted in a fiery peanut sauce with condiments from the island of Java and skewered on thin, wooden sticks.

The chicken is an endless canvas to the chef and a treat to the palate of the eater, especially for the health-conscious. Whether stuffed, minced, grilled or marinated, sweet or sour, pickled or curried, chicken is on menus everywhere.

The versatile chicken is a great dietary ally in maintaining one's weight, and what a source of protein it is! Chicken can be virtually fat-free if the skin is removed prior to cooking or eating. With some creative sauces— sweet or sour, creamed or au jus—you will hardly notice the difference.

The recipes that follow are just the "bare bones" to thousands of other possibilities. After you get the knack of how to "decalorize" your favorite recipe, no doubt you will come up with your own creative culinary masterpiece.

Up, up and away with our friendly bird.

CHICKEN À L'ORANGE

Nutrition Facts
  Number of Servings: 2
  Per Serving
  • Calories: 356
  • Saturated Fat: 5.053 grams
  • Monounsaturated Fat: 3.437 grams
  • Polyunsaturated Fat: 1.352 grams
  • Total Fat: 11.05 grams
  • Percentage of Calories From Fat: 28%

If you have ever tasted duck à l'orange, this dish will remind you of the tangy sweetness. It is one of my children's all-time favorites.

8   oz. uncooked chicken pieces, skin removed
1   tsp. chicken seasoning
¼   tsp. onion powder
1   tbsp. cornstarch
½   cup orange juice
½   tbsp. grated fresh orange rind
2   tbsp. sugar
⅛   tsp. cinnamon
1   tsp. garlic powder
¼   tsp. prepared mustard
½   tsp. orange extract
     Salt and freshly ground pepper
1   tbsp. melted butter

1. Rub the chicken with the chicken seasoning and onion powder. Arrange on aluminum foil in a broiler pan. Broil for about 10 to 12 minutes per side, or until tender and no longer pink inside.
2. Dissolve the cornstarch in the cold orange juice, then add the orange rind, sugar, cinnamon, garlic powder, mustard and extract. Cook over medium heat, stirring constantly, until thickened. Add the salt and pepper to taste.
3. Serve the chicken warm with the sauce poured on top. Dot with the butter.

CHICKEN KIEV

Nutrition Facts
Number of Servings: 1
Per Serving
- Calories: 365
- Saturated Fat: 6.294 grams
- Monounsaturated Fat: 4.013 grams
- Polyunsaturated Fat: 1.403 grams
- Total Fat: 12.91 grams
- Percentage of Calories From Fat: 33%

The classic chicken Kiev is notoriously butter-drenched. This slimmer version will leave you wanting more.

5	oz. boneless chicken breast halves, sliced
2	tsp. chicken seasoning
1/4	tsp. onion powder
3	tbsp. chopped fresh chives
3	tbsp. instant nonfat dry milk
2	tsp. melted butter

1. Using a meat mallet or the handle of a heavy cleaver, pound the chicken slices paper-thin. Sprinkle each side of the cutlets with 1 teaspoon of the chicken seasoning and the onion powder. Sprinkle with the chives.
2. With the chives inside, roll each cutlet lengthwise in a long, tight roll and fasten with toothpicks.
3. Mix the dry milk with the remaining 1 teaspoon chicken seasoning. Roll the chicken in this mixture.
4. Line a small baking dish (barely large enough to hold the rolls side by side) with foil. Add the rolls and 1/4 inch water.
5. Cover the rolls loosely with foil. Bake at 350° for about 15 minutes, or until browned and tender. To prevent drying, don't overbake. Drizzle with the butter.

CROQUETTES DE VOLAILLE

Nutrition Facts
  Number of Servings: 2
  Per Serving
  • Calories: 333
  • Saturated Fat: 4.736 grams
  • Monounsaturated Fat: 3.881 grams
  • Polyunsaturated Fat: 1.538 grams
  • Total Fat: 12.42 grams
  • Percentage of Calories From Fat: 33%

Just a few of these delightful chicken "nuggets" will satisfy your appetite.

2 cups thinly sliced fresh mushrooms
   Freshly ground pepper
   Dash of thyme
3/4 cup minced cooked chicken
2 eggs, 1 beaten and 1 separated
1 slice whole-wheat bread, toasted, dried and
   blended into crumbs
1 tsp. minced fresh parsley
1 tsp. chicken seasoning
1/4 tsp. onion powder
   Instant nonfat dry milk
1 tbsp. cornstarch
1/2 cup evaporated skim milk
   Ground nutmeg
2 tsp. lime or lemon juice

1. Cook the mushrooms by adding 2 tablespoons water, a dash of the pepper and the thyme to a saucepan. Turn the heat to high. Reduce immediately to low and cook for about 7 minutes. Keep warm or reheat and drain when ready to serve.
2. Make the croquettes by mixing the chicken, beaten egg, half of the bread crumbs, parsley, chicken seasoning and onion powder. Form several oval croquettes. Add the dry milk if the croquettes need firming up.
3. Beat the egg white thoroughly but not dry. Evenly roll the croquettes in it.
4. Coat a sheet of aluminum foil with olive oil spray and bake the croquettes at 400° until golden brown, about 10 minutes.
5. In a saucepan make the sauce by dissolving the cornstarch in the cold evaporated milk. Add a pinch of the nutmeg and cook over medium heat, stirring, until thickened. Add the lime or lemon juice and more of the pepper. Keep warm.
6. Just before serving, beat the egg yolk and stir into the sauce. Return to low heat, stirring constantly, just until the egg is cooked. The egg will curdle a bit.
7. Pour this sauce over the croquettes and place the mushrooms around the edge of the plate. Dust with more of the nutmeg, if desired.

CHICKEN CACCIATORE

Nutrition Facts
  Number of Servings: 1
  Per Serving
  • Calories: 424
  • Saturated Fat: 3.095 grams
  • Monounsaturated Fat: 8.835 grams
  • Polyunsaturated Fat: 2.373 grams
  • Total Fat: 16.03 grams
  • Percentage of Calories From Fat: 34%

One of those traditions that should never disappear. The kitchen will evoke the old country's aroma.

5   oz. chicken pieces, skin removed
1   tsp. chicken seasoning
1   cup tomato juice
1   tbsp. minced fresh basil or 1/4 tsp. crumbled dried basil
1   bay leaf, dried
1/2 medium green pepper, cut into strips
1   cup thinly sliced fresh mushrooms or 1/3 cup sliced canned mushrooms
2   cloves garlic, minced
2   tbsp. minced onions
    Salt and freshly ground pepper
2   tsp. olive oil

1. In a nonstick skillet brown the chicken over medium heat by adding 1 to 2 tablespoons water and the chicken seasoning. Turn the chicken in the pan liquid. Add more water if necessary.
2. Add the remaining ingredients except the oil, adding the salt and pepper to taste. If you use the canned mushrooms, wait another 15 minutes before adding them to the liquid.
3. Cover and simmer for about 30 minutes, or until the chicken is tender. Remove the bay leaf. If the liquid is not reduced sufficiently, turn to a higher heat to absorb most of it. Drizzle the oil over the chicken.

A TIP FOR THE COOK

Exercise caution when handling uncooked chicken; chicken often plays host to *Salmonella* germs. Here are some tips:

- Wash your hands before and after handling raw poultry.
- Scrub the countertop, cutting board and cutlery with hot, soapy water after using.
- Thaw chicken in the refrigerator or microwave—not on the counter.
- Refrigerate leftovers within an hour of serving.

SWEET-AND-SOUR GINGERED CHICKEN

Nutrition Facts
  Number of Servings: 1
  Per Serving
  • Calories: 609
  • Saturated Fat: 2.928 grams
  • Monounsaturated Fat: 3.534 grams
  • Polyunsaturated Fat: 2.309 grams
  • Total Fat: 10.42 grams
  • Percentage of Calories From Fat: 15%

Why would anyone go for dessert after this sweet delicacy?

   8   oz. uncooked chicken pieces, skin removed
   2   stalks celery, cut into chunks
  1/4 cup soy sauce
  2 1/2 tbsp. white vinegar
   1   tbsp. honey
  1/2 tsp. grated fresh ginger or 1 tsp. ground ginger
   1   tsp. grated fresh orange rind
  2/3 cup diet pineapple soda or orange soda
  1/4 tsp. pineapple flavoring
   1   tbsp. dried onion flakes

1. Marinate the chicken and celery in the remaining ingredients for 2 hours or overnight in the refrigerator.
2. Remove the celery to a small skillet. Cover with water and simmer, uncovered, until the celery is tender and the liquid is absorbed.
3. Remove the chicken from its marinade and arrange in a baking dish. In a blender jar combine the marinade and celery and whirl until smooth. Cover the chicken with the sauce, then cover with foil.
4. Bake at 350° for about 45 minutes. Remove the foil and bake for about 20 minutes more, or until the chicken is tender.

SPICY CHICKEN

Nutrition Facts
Number of Servings: 1
Per Serving
- Calories: 304
- Saturated Fat: 2.173 grams
- Monounsaturated Fat: 2.632 grams
- Polyunsaturated Fat: 1.672 grams
- Total Fat: 7.988 grams
- Percentage of Calories From Fat: 25%

My children and their young friends loved this preparation. None of them ever knew that their bird had no skin. This version is crispy.

6	oz. uncooked chicken thighs or legs, skin removed
1	tbsp. curry powder (preferably Madras type)
1/4	tsp. (or more) garlic powder
	Ground ginger
	Salt and freshly ground pepper

1. Preheat the oven to 350°.
2. Line a baking pan with aluminum foil and arrange the chicken pieces side by side. Sprinkle each lavishly with the curry, then the garlic powder. Sprinkle lightly with the ginger, salt and pepper.
3. Bake, uncovered, for about 30 minutes. Turn the pieces and season in the same manner. Bake 20 to 30 minutes more, or until a crisp, brown crust has formed.

CHICKEN POLENTA

Nutrition Facts
   Number of Servings: 1
   Per Serving
   • Calories: 486
   • Saturated Fat: 8.537 grams
   • Monounsaturated Fat: 2.374 grams
   • Polyunsaturated Fat: 1.847 grams
   • Total Fat: 8.537 grams
   • Percentage of Calories From Fat: 16%

Long after the cornfields of northern Italy have yielded their golden harvest, polenta remains hardy on the menu. Italian-cut green beans are an excellent accompaniment.

Chicken:
   5   oz. uncooked chicken, skin removed
   1   tsp. chicken seasoning
   3/4   cup tomato sauce
   2   cloves garlic, minced
   1   tbsp. minced fresh basil or 1/2 tsp. crumbled
       dried basil
       Crumbled dried rosemary
   1   medium green pepper, cut into strips
   1/3   cup chopped onions
       Salt and freshly ground pepper

Polenta:
   1/4   tsp. salt
       Dash of cayenne pepper or plenty of freshly
       ground pepper
   1   beef bouillon cube
   3   tbsp. yellow cornmeal

1. To make the chicken: Sprinkle enough water on the chicken so that it can be coated with the chicken seasoning, then turn the chicken in the seasoning until it's coated.
2. Lightly coat just the bottom of a nonstick skillet with olive oil spray. Arrange the chicken in the pan and quickly brown the chicken over medium heat, turning once.
3. Cover the chicken with the remaining ingredients except those for the polenta, adding the salt and pepper to taste. Simmer for 40 minutes, or until the chicken is tender. Add more of the salt and pepper, if desired. Cover and keep warm.
4. To make the polenta: Put 1 cup water and the salt, pepper and bouillon in a saucepan. Bring to a rolling boil. Gradually sprinkle the cornmeal over the water, stirring constantly.
5. When a thick mush forms, remove from the heat and cover. Let sit for 5 to 7 minutes before serving. Top with the chicken.

A TIP FOR THE COOK

How can you tell if the baking powder you have is fresh or stale? Add a teaspoon to a cup of hot water. If it bubbles vigorously, the baking powder is effective.

BOUCHÉES À LA REINE

(CHICKEN À LA KING IN TOASTED CUPS)

Nutrition Facts
 Number of Servings: 2
 Per Serving
 • Calories: 233
 • Saturated Fat: 3.758 grams
 • Monounsaturated Fat: 2.717 grams
 • Polyunsaturated Fat: 0.996 gram
 • Total Fat: 9.157 grams
 • Percentage of Calories From Fat: 35%

These small *bouchées* (mouthfuls) are a Belgian art. They sit, rich and smooth, in their pastry cups like jewels in velvet-lined boxes.

1	slice whole-wheat bread
1	cup sliced fresh mushrooms or ½ cup sliced canned mushrooms, drained (save 1 tbsp. of the liquid)
2	tbsp. minced green onions
	Salt and freshly ground pepper
½	cup evaporated skim milk
1	tbsp. cornstarch
	Pinch of ground nutmeg
¼	tsp. garlic powder
½	cup diced cooked chicken
1	hard-cooked egg, chopped
½	tsp. lime or lemon juice
2	tsp. melted butter

1. With a serrated knife carefully cut the bread in half through its crust to make 2 very thin slices. A very slight toasting will make slicing easier. Slightly dampen the bread with a few drops of water to soften, then roll the bread paper-thin with a rolling pin.
2. Lightly coat custard cups with olive oil spray. Mold each slice of bread into a custard cup or muffin tin to form a cup shape. Reserve.
3. Combine the fresh mushrooms, onions, $1/8$ teaspoon of the salt, pepper to taste and 1 tablespoon water in a saucepan. Cover and place over high heat. Immediately turn down the heat to the lowest possible setting and cook for 10 minutes. If canned mushrooms are used, simmer for 5 minutes in the reserved liquid with the onions and the pepper but without the salt. Drain the mushrooms and reserve.
4. Put the milk in a small saucepan and dissolve the cornstarch. Add the nutmeg and garlic powder. Cook over medium heat, stirring constantly, until thickened.
5. Add the chicken, eggs, mushroom mixture, lime or lemon juice and more of the salt and pepper to taste. Remove from the heat and keep warm.
6. Bake the toasted cups at 350° until golden brown, about 10 minutes. Fill the cups and drizzle the butter over the tops. Remove the toasted cups from their cups or tins and arrange on a serving platter.

WATERZOOI KIEKEN

Nutrition Facts
Number of Servings: 4
Per Serving
- Calories: 400
- Saturated Fat: 1.645 grams
- Monounsaturated Fat: 1.827 grams
- Polyunsaturated Fat: 1.624 grams
- Total Fat: 6.22 grams
- Percentage of Calories From Fat: 14%

For those days when a return to simple, homey flavors is welcome. I like this stew over crisp brown rice for contrast.

1	lb. chicken pieces, skin removed
8	stalks celery, minced
3–4	leeks, chopped (white part only)
1½–2	cups chopped green onions (including tops)
2	chicken bouillon cubes
¼	cup fresh minced parsley
	Bouquet garni of 2 crushed dried bay leaves, 10 whole black peppercorns and 5 whole cloves, tied in cheesecloth or placed in a metal tea ball
1	tbsp. fresh dill or 1 tsp. dried dill
1	tsp. ground sage
1	tsp. dried thyme
	Salt and freshly ground pepper
¼	cup evaporated skim milk
1	tbsp. dry white wine or brandy flavoring (if desired)

1. In a large saucepan arrange the chicken, celery, leeks, onions and bouillon. Add water to about the halfway point of the vegetables and chicken.
2. Add the herbs and spices and the salt and pepper to taste. Bring to a boil, cover and simmer over low heat for about 45 minutes, or until the chicken pulls away from the bones. Check the water often to end up with a much-reduced bouillon. Remove the bouquet garni.
3. At serving time stir in the milk, wine or flavoring (if using) and more of the salt if necessary.

MEATS

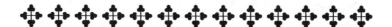

One of the secrets of changing one's lifelong eating habits is to not go "cold turkey" on meat—particularly today, when so many low-fat meats can be found at your supermarket. Take, for instance, hamburger meat. It comes in a variety of lowered fat counts, as low as 90 percent fat-free. My family and I spent hours in Cairo, Egypt, looking for a hamburger place for our children. After weeks of traveling they both felt horribly homesick without hamburgers. We ended up eating camelburgers. They were delicious, and somehow they did the trick.

And speaking of cold turkey, another new product is becoming increasingly popular in the United States: ground turkey! Ground turkey is so "docile" that it will take on any flavor you give to it. And what a source of low-fat protein it is.

The little pig has gone on a diet, too. Some pork cutlets are virtually fat-free. Or you can remove all visible fat before cooking.

When it comes to lamb, I am definitely a fanatic. Whether you prepare moussaka (recipe on page 134) or stuffed cabbage rolls (recipe on page 138), they are succulent, "decalorized" versions of the real ones.

And now for a quick lamb barbecue: Remove the visible fat from a leg of lamb and cube the meat. Prepare a marinade of red wine, minced fresh basil, crumbled oregano, vinegar, dried bay leaves, ground cumin and tons and tons of garlic. Marinate overnight. Skewer the cubes on wooden or other skewers (remember to soak wooden ones in water to prevent burning). Arrange green pepper slices, mushrooms and onion chunks between the lamb pieces. And barbecue! Or cook in your regular broiler.

SWEET-AND-SOUR MEATBALLS

Nutrition Facts
  Number of Servings: 2
  Per Serving
  • Calories: 332
  • Saturated Fat: 4.061 grams
  • Monounsaturated Fat: 4.304 grams
  • Polyunsaturated Fat: 0.571 gram
  • Total Fat: 10.3 grams
  • Percentage of Calories From Fat: 28%

Wide noodles or brown rice is a delicious accompaniment to this sweet-and-sour dish.

1/2	cup unsweetened crushed pineapple, drained (save the juice)
1	stalk celery, minced
1	tbsp. low-sodium soy sauce
1	tsp. vinegar
1	tsp. grated fresh ginger or 1/4 tsp. ground ginger
2	tbsp. sugar
1/4	lb. extra-lean ground beef
1/4	lb. ground turkey breast
1/4	tsp. onion powder
1/4	tsp. garlic powder
1/3	cup instant nonfat dry milk
	Salt and freshly ground pepper
1/2	green pepper, cut into 3/4-inch pieces

1. In a skillet combine several tablespoons of the pineapple juice and the celery and simmer, adding more of the juice if necessary, just until the celery is tender.
2. Drain and add the soy sauce, vinegar, ginger, sugar and pineapple. Simmer for a few minutes until some of the liquid has evaporated. Cover and remove from the heat. Reserve.
3. In a mixing bowl combine the beef, turkey, onion powder, garlic powder, dry milk and salt and pepper to taste. Mix well and form into small meatballs, adding water if necessary to obtain firm yet still moist balls.
4. Alternately skewer the meatballs with the green pepper pieces. If wooden skewers are used, soak them in water first to prevent burning. Arrange the skewers on a broiler rack and broil for 5 minutes on each side, or until the meat is no longer pink inside.
5. Reheat the sauce and pour over the meatballs. Serve at once.

GRINGO ENCHILADAS

Nutrition Facts
  Number of Servings: 4
  Per Serving
  • Calories: 361
  • Saturated Fat: 4.419 grams
  • Monounsaturated Fat: 6.131 grams
  • Polyunsaturated Fat: 1.111 grams
  • Total Fat: 13.9 grams
  • Percentage of Calories From Fat: 34%

The Ortegas in Taxco, Mexico, were baffled by this copy-cat wrapper containing the original rich Mexican flavors. Gloria ate two servings. Olé!

1/2	lb. extra-lean ground beef
1/2	lb. ground turkey breast
1/2	tsp. onion powder
1–2	tbsp. chili powder
4	cloves garlic, minced
1/4	cup low-sodium tomato sauce
1/8	tsp. ground cumin
	Freshly ground pepper
1	cup canned kidney beans, drained
4	slices whole-wheat bread
	Paprika
2	tsp. olive oil

1. In a bowl combine the beef, turkey and onion powder and mix well. Form into 2 thin patties and broil on each side until the fat has dripped out but the meat is still moist.
2. Crumble the meat with a fork while it is still warm and drain any remaining fat. Add the chili powder, garlic, tomato sauce, cumin and pepper to taste. Mix.
3. In a blender jar puree the beans until smooth. Add to the meat mixture and adjust the seasonings. Reserve for the filling.
4. Lightly sprinkle paprika on both sides of the bread. With a rolling pin roll each slice as thin as possible without tearing.
5. In the center of each wrapper spoon a quarter of the meat mixture. Fold the bread over to form a triangle-shaped turnover and seal the edges by moistening them with water and pressing around them with fork tines.
6. With a spatula arrange the enchiladas on a baking sheet and bake, uncovered, at 350° for 15 minutes, or until toasted and hot. Drizzle with the oil. Serve warm and crisp.

VEAL PAUPIETTES

Nutrition Facts
  Number of Servings: 2
  Per Serving
  • Calories: 235
  • Saturated Fat: 2.728 grams
  • Monounsaturated Fat: 2.324 grams
  • Polyunsaturated Fat: 0.718 gram
  • Total Fat: 7.101 grams
  • Percentage of Calories From Fat: 27%

For a variation try this with chicken breast cutlets. Goes well with brown rice or noodles.

1 1/3 cups chopped fresh mushrooms or 1/2 cup minced canned mushrooms, drained
        Salt
8   oz. veal, thinly sliced (as for veal scaloppine)
2   tsp. chicken seasoning
1   slice whole-wheat or multigrain bread, toasted, dried and blended into fine crumbs
1   tsp. minced fresh parsley or 1/2 tsp. dried parsley
1/2   tbsp. minced fresh garlic or 1/4 tsp. garlic powder
        Freshly ground pepper
        Crumbled dried thyme
2   oz. onion, chopped
2   oz. carrot, diced
1/2   tsp. sherry or wine flavoring (if desired)
        Lime juice
1/2   tsp. butter

1. Simmer the fresh mushrooms in 2 tablespoons water and ¼ teaspoon of the salt for about 7 minutes. Drain and reserve.
2. Place the veal between 2 layers of waxed paper and pound until thin.
3. In a bowl combine the cooked or canned mushrooms, 1 teaspoon of the chicken seasoning, bread crumbs, parsley, garlic or garlic powder and pepper and more of the salt to taste. Divide this mixture evenly onto each cutlet and roll tightly. Tie with white cotton string. Sprinkle the rolls lightly with the thyme.
4. Sprinkle the remaining 1 teaspoon chicken seasoning onto the rolls. In a saucepan add just enough water so that the seasoning adheres to the rolls as you turn them, searing them. Do this until the rolls are slightly browned. When browned, add ½ cup water and the onions and carrots.
5. Cover and barely simmer for 30 minutes, or until most of the liquid is gone (if you need more water, add it 1 spoonful at a time). Pour the flavoring over the rolls, cover and simmer for 1 minute longer.
6. When ready to serve, drizzle with the lime juice to taste and dot with the butter. Eat warm.

VEAL PARMIGIANA

Nutrition Facts
Number of Servings: 1
Per Serving
- Calories: 216
- Saturated Fat: 3.402 grams
- Monounsaturated Fat: 2.307 grams
- Polyunsaturated Fat: 0.406 gram
- Total Fat: 6.949 grams
- Percentage of Calories From Fat: 29%

Lean, lean is the veal, yet this preparation makes it taste sinfully rich. Excellent with noodles or rice.

3	oz. veal, thinly sliced (as for veal scaloppine)
1	tsp. chicken seasoning
1/4	tsp. onion powder
1/3	cup tomato sauce or puree
1	tbsp. minced fresh parsley or 1 tsp. dried parsley
1/4 – 1/2 tsp.	garlic powder
1/4	tsp. crumbled dried rosemary
1/4	tsp. crumbled oregano
	Freshly ground pepper
2	tbsp. low-fat mozzarella cheese
1	tbsp. Parmesan cheese

1. Place the veal between 2 layers of waxed paper and pound until thin. Sprinkle each side with the chicken seasoning and onion powder. Place in a baking dish in a single layer.
2. In a bowl combine the tomato sauce or puree, parsley, garlic powder, rosemary, oregano and pepper to taste. Spread half of this over the meat and top with the mozzarella. Spread the remaining sauce mixture over the cheese layer. Sprinkle with the Parmesan.
3. Bake at 350° for about 20 to 25 minutes, adding a spoonful of water at a time, if necessary, to keep the veal moist. Eat warm.

YOGURT KABOBS

Nutrition Facts
Number of Servings: 2
Per Serving
- Calories: 302
- Saturated Fat: 3.962 grams
- Monounsaturated Fat: 4.782 grams
- Polyunsaturated Fat: 0.725 gram
- Total Fat: 11.23 grams
- Percentage of Calories From Fat: 34%

Once upon a time the "yogurtly" kabob was prepared with all of the spices this version contains. Nowadays modern chefs have simplified the preparation. So here's to bygone days. Quick, too.

8	oz. lean lamb, ground
1	tsp. ground cumin
1/2	tsp. ground coriander
1/4	tsp. ground turmeric
1/4	tsp. ground cardamom
	Several dashes of cinnamon
	Salt and freshly ground pepper
3–4	cloves garlic, minced
1	beef bouillon cube
3/4	cup plain low-fat yogurt

1. In a bowl mix the lamb with the spices, adding the salt and pepper to taste. Shape into small meatballs and put on a rack in a broiler pan. Broil, turning, until browned but still very moist.
2. In a skillet combine 1/4 cup water and the garlic and bouillon and bring to a boil. Add the meatballs, lower the heat and simmer until the water is absorbed, about 12 to 14 minutes. Cool slightly.
3. Add the yogurt. Heat, stirring, just until hot. Do not let it boil, or the sauce will curdle.

BARBECUED BEEF RIBS

Nutrition Facts
  Number of Servings: 6
  Per Serving
  • Calories: 307
  • Saturated Fat: 4.6 grams
  • Monounsaturated Fat: 4.786 grams
  • Polyunsaturated Fat: 0.362 gram
  • Total Fat: 11.54 grams
  • Percentage of Calories From Fat: 35%

Beef ribs are not like pork or lamb ribs; they are fairly lean, and the meat is so tender that it can be broiled.

12	beef ribs
6	cloves garlic, pureed
1/4	cup low-sodium soy sauce
1/2	tsp. ground ginger
3/4	cup white wine vinegar
10	whole black peppercorns
2	dried bay leaves
1/3	cup brown sugar
2/3	cup instant nonfat dry milk
1	cup unsweetened crushed pineapple, drained

1. Lay the ribs side by side in a marinade dish.
2. In a saucepan combine the remaining ingredients except the dry milk and pineapple. Bring to a boil and pour over the ribs. Cover with foil and refrigerate overnight, turning occasionally.
3. Drain and reserve the marinade. Remove the bay leaves.
4. Coat only 1 side of the ribs with half of the dry milk and arrange milk side up on a broiler rack. Broil for 12 to 15 minutes, basting occasionally with the marinade. Turn the ribs and coat the other side with the remaining dry milk. Broil for 10 minutes.
5. Spread the pineapple evenly over the top and return to the broiler just until the fruit is browned and forms a varnish that bubbles and adheres to the ribs. Don't cook beyond medium-rare, or the meat will toughen.

TAMALE PIE

Nutrition Facts
Number of Servings: 2
Per Serving
- Calories: 358
- Saturated Fat: 4.338 grams
- Monounsaturated Fat: 5.981 grams
- Polyunsaturated Fat: 0.852 gram
- Total Fat: 13.19 grams
- Percentage of Calories From Fat: 34%

This favorite is a cobbler with a cornmeal crust.

¼	lb. lean ground beef
¼	lb. ground turkey breast
½	tsp. onion powder
⅔	cup low-sodium tomato sauce
1–2	tbsp. chili powder
2	cloves garlic, minced
½	medium onion, sliced into thin rings
1	beef bouillon cube
1	medium green pepper, cut into strips
3	tbsp. yellow cornmeal
1	tsp. olive oil

1. Mix the beef, turkey and onion powder. Shape into a thin patty. Broil on each side until the fat has dripped out but the meat is still moist. Crumble with a fork while warm and drain any remaining fat.
2. In a bowl mix the meat with the tomato sauce, chili powder and garlic. Spread the mixture evenly in a baking dish. Top with the onions. Reserve.
3. Put the bouillon and 1 cup plus 2 tablespoons water into a skillet. Bring to a boil and blanch the peppers until tender-crisp. Remove with a slotted spoon and arrange the strips on top of the onions.
4. Reduce the heat so that the remaining bouillon simmers. Gradually pour in the cornmeal, stirring constantly, and cook until quite thickened. Spread this mixture evenly across the top of the baking dish, sealing the edges.
5. Bake, uncovered, at 350° for 20 to 30 minutes, or until lightly browned on top. Drizzle with the oil.

Meats
❖
131

BLANQUETTE DE VEAU

Nutrition Facts
  Number of Servings: 2
  Per Serving
  • Calories: 265
  • Saturated Fat: 4.335 grams
  • Monounsaturated Fat: 2.861 grams
  • Polyunsaturated Fat: 0.612 gram
  • Total Fat: 8.927 grams
  • Percentage of Calories From Fat: 30%

This dish is the aristocrat of stews! Great served over brown rice or large noodles.

1	tsp. chicken seasoning
7	oz. boneless lean veal, cubed
1/2	medium onion, sliced into thin rings
1/3	cup thinly sliced carrots
	Bouquet garni of 1 dried bay leaf, 3 whole cloves and 5 whole black peppercorns, tied in cheesecloth or placed in a metal tea ball
2	cloves garlic, minced
1	cup sliced fresh mushrooms or 1/3 cup sliced canned mushrooms
	Salt and freshly ground pepper
1	tbsp. cornstarch
1/2	cup evaporated skim milk
	Pinch of ground nutmeg
1/2	tsp. sherry or wine flavoring (if desired)
1–2	tsp. lime or lemon juice
2	tsp. butter

1. Sprinkle the chicken seasoning onto the veal. In a nonstick skillet over medium heat add just enough water so that the seasoning adheres to the meat as you turn it, searing it. Do this until the meat is slightly browned.
2. Add the onions, carrots, bouquet garni and garlic. Cover with water. Simmer, covered, for 1 hour.
3. Add the mushrooms and the salt and pepper to taste. Simmer, covered, for 1 more hour. The liquid should be reduced to $1/2$ cup. Remove the bouquet garni. Drain the liquid and pour into a small saucepan.
4. Dissolve the cornstarch in the cold milk with the nutmeg and add to the saucepan liquid. Cook over medium heat until thickened, stirring constantly.
5. Add the flavoring if using, lime or lemon juice and more of the salt and pepper if necessary. Pour this sauce over the veal and vegetables and drizzle with the butter. The result should be a creamy white, almost transparent stew.

A TIP FOR THE COOK

What can you do when you've scorched the rice, and there's no time to make more? Scoop the rice into a clean pot, being careful not to include the blackened bottom part. Place a layer of onion skins—the first few layers of the onion, minus the papery part—over the rice and cover. The skins will absorb the smoky taste in about 10 minutes.

MOUSSAKA

Nutrition Facts
Number of Servings: 2
Per Serving
- Calories: 418
- Saturated Fat: 4.961 grams
- Monounsaturated Fat: 6.766 grams
- Polyunsaturated Fat: 1.049 grams
- Total Fat: 14.55 grams
- Percentage of Calories From Fat: 31%

No Greek gathering goes without this elegant casserole.
Make ahead of time and reheat before serving.

2	small eggplants
	Salt
8	oz. lean lamb, ground
1	tsp. chicken seasoning
1	tbsp. minced onions
2	cloves garlic, minced
2/3	cup tomato sauce or puree
1	tbsp. minced fresh parsley
1/4	tsp. sherry or wine flavoring (if desired)
1/8	tsp. cinnamon
	Ground nutmeg
	Freshly ground pepper
1	tbsp. cornstarch
3/4	cup evaporated skim milk
1	tbsp. grated Parmesan cheese
1	tsp. olive oil

1. Cut the eggplants lengthwise into thin slices. Lightly sprinkle both sides with the salt and put on plenty of paper towels to let the water and bitter flavor come out.
2. Wipe off the remaining salt and drop the slices into boiling water, cooking until just tender. Dry on paper towels.
3. Mix the lamb with the chicken seasoning, onions and garlic and shape into a thin patty. Broil on both sides on a broiler rack until the fat has dripped out but the meat is still moist.
4. Crumble the warm meat in a bowl and drain any remaining fat. Add $^1/_3$ cup of the tomato sauce or puree and the parsley, flavoring if using, cinnamon, a pinch of the nutmeg, and pepper and more of the salt to taste.
5. In a 9-inch baking pan, layer half of the eggplant, then the lamb mixture and the remaining eggplant over the top. Pour the remaining $^1/_3$ cup tomato sauce over it.
6. Dissolve the cornstarch into the cold milk, add a pinch of the nutmeg and cook in a small saucepan over medium heat until thickened. Pour this creamed sauce over the moussaka. Sprinkle evenly with the cheese and bake at 350° for 20 to 30 minutes, or until hot and browned. Drizzle with the oil.

LULEH KABOB

Nutrition Facts
   Number of Servings: 1
   Per Serving
   • Calories: 468
   • Saturated Fat: 6.536 grams
   • Monounsaturated Fat: 7.492 grams
   • Polyunsaturated Fat: 1.347 grams
   • Total Fat: 17.97 grams
   • Percentage of Calories From Fat: 34%

This delicious dish is seasoned exotically, and the spiced meatballs are skewered with fresh vegetable chunks. Serve over brown rice or couscous.

6	oz. lean lamb, ground
1/4	tsp. onion powder
1/4	tsp. ground cumin
1/4	tsp. cinnamon
3/4	tsp. crumbled dried mint leaves
	Salt and freshly ground pepper
1	medium firm tomato, chunked
1	medium green pepper, cut into square pieces
1/2	cup buttermilk
1	beef bouillon cube
1/4	tsp. ground coriander
1/2	tsp. minced fresh parsley or 1/4 tsp. dried parsley
1	tbsp. lemon juice

1. In a bowl mix the lamb, onion powder, cumin, cinnamon, 1/2 teaspoon of the mint and the salt and ground pepper to taste. Shape into 9 meatballs.
2. Skewer kabobs by alternating the meatballs with the tomatoes and green peppers. If wooden skewers are used, soak them in water first to prevent burning. Place on a broiler rack and broil until browned and no longer pink inside.
3. In a small skillet combine the remaining ingredients. Heat through. Do not let it boil, or the sauce will curdle. Pour over the skewers.

MALAYSIAN KABOBS

Nutrition Facts
Number of Servings: 2
Per Serving
- Calories: 271
- Saturated Fat: 2.126 grams
- Monounsaturated Fat: 1.542 grams
- Polyunsaturated Fat: 1.128 grams
- Total Fat: 6.983 grams
- Percentage of Calories From Fat: 23%

For us liver-haters this dish is a sure way to conversion.

8	oz. chicken livers, cut into pieces
1/4	cup low-sodium soy sauce
1/2	green pepper, cut into 1-inch pieces
1	cup small mushrooms or large ones cut in half
1/2	cup unsweetened pineapple chunks (save 2 tbsp. of the juice)
1/8	tsp. turmeric or curry powder
1	tsp. grated fresh ginger or 1/8 tsp. ground ginger
1/4	tsp. garlic powder
	Freshly ground pepper
2	tsp. brown sugar

1. Lightly coat a nonstick skillet with olive oil spray.
2. Fry the liver in just a little of the soy sauce and enough water to make a glaze that promotes browning. Cook until firm but still pink inside.
3. Skewer kabobs by alternating the liver, peppers, mushrooms and pineapple. If wooden skewers are used, soak them in water first to prevent burning.
4. Arrange the kabobs side by side in a broiler pan lined with aluminum foil. Brush the kabobs with the remaining soy sauce and the pineapple juice. Sprinkle evenly with the turmeric or curry powder, ginger, garlic powder and lots of the ground pepper to taste.
5. Broil for 5 minutes on each side, or until the vegetables are tender-crisp and the liver is no longer pink inside. Add the brown sugar to the pan liquid and serve as a sauce over the kabobs.

STUFFED CABBAGE ROLLS

Nutrition Facts
Number of Servings: 2
Per Serving
- Calories: 419
- Saturated Fat: 4.066 grams
- Monounsaturated Fat: 4.989 grams
- Polyunsaturated Fat: 1.28 grams
- Total Fat: 12.21 grams
- Percentage of Calories From Fat: 25%

This generous portion seems to contain mega-fat and calories. Surprise: It is lean, lean, lean. This is hearty, delicious home-cooked fare.

1	medium head cabbage
8	oz. lean lamb, ground
1	tbsp. minced onions
2	tsp. minced fresh mint leaves or 1 tsp. dried mint
1/4	tsp. cinnamon
1/4	tsp. ground cumin
2	cloves garlic, minced
1	firm tomato, finely chopped
1/2	cup cooked brown rice
1	cup tomato juice
1	tbsp. lemon juice
1	beef bouillon cube
	Salt and freshly ground pepper

1. Prepare the cabbage by discarding the outer leaves. Immerse the head in boiling water until the leaves pull off easily and are somewhat flexible. Drain thoroughly.
2. In a mixing bowl combine the lamb, onions, half of the mint, cinnamon, cumin and half of the garlic. Form into a thin patty and arrange on a broiler rack. Broil on either side just until the fat has been rendered but the meat is still moist.
3. Crumble the meat with a fork while warm. Mix in the chopped tomatoes and rice.
4. Shape the rolls, with the cabbage leaves serving as wrappers. Start with the smaller leaves and cut the larger leaves to size. Place a spoonful of the lamb filling in the center of each leaf. Fold the ends in over the filling, then fold 1 side over and roll up. Fasten with toothpicks.
5. Arrange the rolls side by side in a larger skillet. Pour the tomato juice and lemon juice over the rolls. Add the bouillon and the remaining mint and garlic and the salt and pepper to taste. Put a heavy plate on top of the rolls to prevent unrolling.
6. Cover and simmer for 20 minutes, or until a thick sauce has formed. Serve and eat hot.

PORK SATÉ

Nutrition Facts
  Number of Servings: 6
  Per Serving
  • Calories: 285
  • Saturated Fat: 1.745 grams
  • Monounsaturated Fat: 2.895 grams
  • Polyunsaturated Fat: 2.287 grams
  • Total Fat: 7.98 grams
  • Percentage of Calories From Fat: 25%

We enjoyed such aromatic fare broiled over charcoal right at our table in Singapore's famous "Car-Park." The smell is enough to awaken any appetite.

1	lb. 12 oz. boneless pork tenderloin, cut into 1-inch cubes
2–3	cups small mushrooms or larger ones cut in half (should be about 1 inch in diameter)
1	lb. small onions (the size of walnuts)
3	tbsp. low-sodium soy sauce
1/4	cup white wine vinegar
1	tbsp. minced garlic
1	tsp. turmeric or curry powder
	Freshly ground pepper
2	tbsp. low-calorie mayonnaise
1	cup canned chickpeas, or garbanzo beans, drained (save the liquid)
2	tbsp. brown sugar
1	tbsp. sesame oil or peanut butter (I like peanut butter in this recipe.)
1	tsp. walnut or peanut flavoring (if desired)
	Hot pepper sauce

1. In a large bowl combine the pork, mushrooms and onions.
2. In a saucepan combine $1/2$ cup water and the soy sauce, vinegar, garlic, turmeric or curry powder and pepper to taste and bring to a boil. Pour over the pork and vegetables and marinate for several hours, or preferably overnight in the refrigerator. Turn the pieces occasionally.
3. Skewer the meat on wooden or other skewers by alternating the vegetables and pork. If wooden skewers are used, soak them in water first to prevent burning.
4. Arrange the skewers on a broiler rack and broil, turning and basting occasionally with marinade. Or charcoal broil. The pork should be thoroughly cooked and no longer pink inside. Do not overcook, so as not to toughen the meat.
5. In a blender jar combine the remaining ingredients, including the flavoring if using, and adding the hot pepper sauce to taste. Blend until smooth, adding the chickpea liquid as necessary. Heat this mixture in a saucepan and pour it over the kabobs.

PASTITSIO

Nutrition Facts
Number of Servings: 2
Per Serving
- Calories: 386
- Saturated Fat: 4.158 grams
- Monounsaturated Fat: 4.355 grams
- Polyunsaturated Fat: 0.656 gram
- Total Fat: 11.12 grams
- Percentage of Calories From Fat: 26%

A popular buffet dish. Kids love it, too.

1/3	cup uncooked orzo or small macaroni
1/4	lb. extra-lean ground beef
1/4	lb. ground turkey breast
1/3	cup finely chopped onions
2	cloves garlic, minced
2/3	cup low-sodium tomato sauce
1	tbsp. chopped fresh parsley or 1 tsp. dried parsley
1/4	tsp. sherry flavoring (if desired)
	Cinnamon
	Salt and freshly ground pepper
2	tsp. cornstarch
1/3	cup evaporated skim milk
	Ground nutmeg
1	tbsp. instant nonfat dry milk

1. Cook the pasta al dente in boiling salted water. Drain and reserve.
2. Lightly coat a 4-cup baking dish with olive oil spray. Line with half of the cooked pasta. Reserve the remaining pasta.
3. In a bowl mix the beef, turkey and onions and form into a thin patty. Put the patty on a broiler rack and broil until the fat has been rendered but the meat is still moist.
4. While the meat is warm, crumble it with a fork and mix with the garlic, tomato sauce, parsley, flavoring if using, 1/4 teaspoon of the cinnamon and salt and pepper to taste. Spread this mixture evenly across the pasta in the baking dish and cover with the remaining pasta.
5. Dissolve the cornstarch in the cold evaporated milk with a dash of the nutmeg. In a small saucepan over medium heat, bring to a boil, stirring until thickened. Remove from the heat and stir in the dry milk. Spread evenly on the pasta in the baking dish and sprinkle delicately with more of the cinnamon and nutmeg.
6. Bake, uncovered, at 350° for 25 to 30 minutes, or until crusty. If necessary, cover to avoid drying. Let it sit for a few minutes before cutting.

STUFFED ONIONS

Nutrition Facts
  Number of Servings: 3
  Per Serving
  • Calories: 475
  • Saturated Fat: 5.259 grams
  • Monounsaturated Fat: 6.418 grams
  • Polyunsaturated Fat: 1.216 grams
  • Total Fat: 15.14 grams
  • Percentage of Calories From Fat: 29%

An alternative for this hearty preparation would be green or red peppers. Large mushrooms work as well.

1	lb. lean lamb, ground (leg or loin)
1	tbsp. minced onions
1/4	tsp. ground cumin
1/8	tsp. ground coriander
1	tbsp. minced fresh parsley or 1 tsp. dried parsley
1/4	tsp. crumbled dried basil
	Pinch of dried oregano
	Pinch of dried thyme
2	cloves garlic, minced
	Salt and freshly ground pepper
1/4	cup tomato sauce or puree
6	large onions
	Cinnamon

1. In a bowl combine the lamb, minced onions, spices, herbs, garlic and salt and pepper to taste; mix well. Shape into 2 thin patties and put on a broiler rack. Broil on both sides until the fat has rendered but the meat is still moist. Crumble the warm meat with a fork and mix with the tomato sauce or puree.
2. Cut the tops off the whole onions and reserve. Remove enough of the insides to make a thick shell for the stuffing.
3. In a shallow skillet bring 1 inch water to a boil. Immerse the onions side by side in the boiling water and simmer, covered, for about 10 minutes, or until tender but still firm.
4. With a slotted spoon remove the onions from the water. Fill the insides of the onions with the stuffing, packing it tightly to prevent the stuffing from coming out while baking.
5. Arrange in a tight-fitting baking dish, put the caps on and dust delicately with the cinnamon. Add 1 inch hot water and bake at 400° for 20 to 25 minutes, or until the onions are tender and the tops are browned. Cover with aluminum foil if the onions brown too rapidly. Baste often with the pan liquid.

OSSO BUCO

Nutrition Facts
Number of Servings: 2
Per Serving
- Calories: 187
- Saturated Fat: 1.915 grams
- Monounsaturated Fat: 3.158 grams
- Polyunsaturated Fat: 0.573 gram
- Total Fat: 6.444 grams
- Percentage of Calories From Fat: 31%

A filling meal from the Lombardy region of Italy.

8	oz. veal shank or shoulder blade
1	tsp. chicken seasoning
1/2	medium onion, thinly sliced
1/3	cup finely chopped carrots
1	stalk celery, minced
2	tsp. minced fresh parsley
1/8	tsp. oregano
2	cloves garlic, minced
1	dried bay leaf
	Freshly ground pepper
1	cup low-sodium tomato juice
1	tsp. grated lemon rind
1/2	tsp. sherry flavoring (if desired)
1	tsp. olive oil

1. In a nonstick skillet over medium-high heat sprinkle the veal with the chicken seasoning. Add just enough water so that the seasoning sticks to the meat as you turn it, searing it. Do this until the meat is slightly browned.
2. Top with the onions, carrots, celery, parsley, oregano, garlic and bay leaf. Add the pepper to taste. Slowly pour the tomato juice over top, not disturbing the vegetables.
3. Cover the dish and simmer for about 1 1/4 hours, adding water if necessary. When the meat pulls away from the bones and the liquid is thickened to a puree, the dish is ready to be served. Remove the bay leaf.
4. Add the lemon rind and flavoring if using. Pour the oil over top.

SAVORY SWEETS
AND DESSERTS

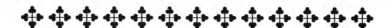

Fresh, sun-ripened fruit is the dessert par excellence. We are told to eat at least two to four pieces of fruit a day. But because some of us crave "real" desserts, I have put together some of these sweet treats combining the natural flavor of fruit with just a touch of honey or sugar. Some of these treats can be eaten for breakfast instead of your regular breakfast. Because of their bulk and fiber content, they are very satisfying.

Create your own desserts using the simple methods described in my recipes. My daughter Tatiana's favorite dessert/luncheon used to be a mixture of 1 cup of frozen strawberries, 2/3 cup of low-fat cottage cheese or low-fat ricotta cheese, some cinnamon and 1 to 2 tablespoons of sugar. She whirled these together in a blender jar, and presto! She had a creamy, velvety, frozen dessert so satisfying that she needed nothing else for that meal.

Try toasting two pieces of whole-grain bread. Spread 2/3 cup of low-fat ricotta cheese evenly on top. Divide 1 cup of sliced strawberries and arrange the fruit on top of the cheese. Sprinkle delicately with cinnamon and 1 to 2 tablespoons of sugar. Arrange on a nonstick oven plate and bake for a few minutes. It will be thick and taste like a cream-cheese cake!

For a different sweet treat: Scoop out and shape some melon balls and freeze. Eat frozen, dusted with ground ginger. Or sprinkle a banana with a touch of sugar and ginger or cinnamon. Freeze on a wooden ice-cream stick and eat. These are only some ideas among hundreds. The sky is the limit—and then some.

BLANCMANGE WITH BERRIES

Nutrition Facts
Number of Servings: 2
Per Serving
- Calories: 336
- Saturated Fat: 0.344 gram
- Monounsaturated Fat: 0.261 gram
- Polyunsaturated Fat: 0.299 gram
- Total Fat: 1.102 grams
- Percentage of Calories From Fat: 3%

This sweet, creamy treat can accommodate any fresh fruit or berry. Here is another way to drink your milk and eat your fruit, too. Look at the calorie count and the fat content! Enjoy without guilt.

1   envelope unflavored gelatin
2   cups evaporated skim milk
3   tbsp. sugar
    Almond extract
2   cups sliced fresh strawberries, chilled

1. In a saucepan soften the gelatin in the cold milk and cook over low heat, stirring constantly.
2. When the gelatin is dissolved, remove from the heat and stir in the sugar. Add the extract a drop at a time to taste.
3. Pour into individual custard cups, 2 1-cup molds or a bowl. Chill until very firm.
4. When ready to serve, dip the dish in warm water for a few seconds and unmold onto a serving plate. Top or surround with the strawberries. If using individual custard cups, there is no need to unmold. Just top with the fruit and spoon right out of the cup.

CREAMY BANANA MOLD

Nutrition Facts
  Number of Servings: 2
  Per Serving
  • Calories: 141
  • Saturated Fat: 0.126 gram
  • Monounsaturated Fat: 0.045 gram
  • Polyunsaturated Fat: 0.075 gram
  • Total Fat: 0.409 gram
  • Percentage of Calories From Fat: 2%

You could replace the banana with a peach, an apricot or even one of those jams sweetened with natural fruit juices. Your choice.

1	medium very ripe banana, peeled and mashed
2	tbsp. uncooked Cream of Wheat cereal (farina)
	Tiny pinch of salt
2	tbsp. sugar
½	tsp. banana or rum flavoring (if desired)
	Pinch of mace or ground nutmeg

1. Combine the mashed banana and ¾ cup water in a small skillet. Bring to a boil and gradually sprinkle in the farina in a steady stream, stirring constantly. Cook for 2 minutes, or until thickened and smooth, making sure no clumps form.
2. Remove from the heat and immediately stir in the remaining ingredients including the flavoring if using. Cover and let stand for a few minutes.
3. Stir and pour into 2 individual custard cups or a small bowl. Chill until firm.
4. Spoon right out of the cup or bowl or unmold by dipping the bottom into hot water for a few seconds. The cooler this treat is, the better it tastes.

Savory
Sweets
and
Desserts
❖
149

APPLE CAKE

Nutrition Facts

Number of Servings: 6

Per Serving
- Calories: 193
- Saturated Fat: 0.648 gram
- Monounsaturated Fat: 2.312 grams
- Polyunsaturated Fat: 2.12 grams
- Total Fat: 5.455 grams
- Percentage of Calories From Fat: 25%

One of these wedges will make do for a dessert or a whole breakfast, fruit and all.

4	medium juicy, sweet apples, cored
1	cup fat-free egg substitute
2	egg whites (for added moistness)
4	slices white bread, toasted and torn into pieces
3/4	tsp. baking soda
1/8	tsp. cream of tartar
4	tbsp. sugar
2	tbsp. applesauce
2	tbsp. sunflower oil
	Almond extract
	Cinnamon

1. Cut the apples in half horizontally, through their sides. Arrange the apple halves side by side in a 10-inch skillet, adding 1/2 inch water. Cover and simmer the apples until soft but still standing upright.
2. With a slotted spoon carefully remove the apples. Drain them and put them side by side in a 9-inch pie plate.
3. In a blender jar combine the egg substitute, egg whites, bread, baking soda, cream of tartar, sugar, applesauce and oil. Blend until smooth, adding the extract a drop at a time to taste. Pour this batter over the apples to fill the empty spaces.
4. Bake, uncovered, at 350° for about 20 minutes, or until browned and cakelike. Cover if it is browning too fast.
5. Remove from the oven and sprinkle lightly with the cinnamon. Eat warm or cold.

HUNGARY

CRUSTY APPLE PIE

Nutrition Facts
Number of Servings: 6
Per Serving
- Calories: 302
- Saturated Fat: 0.998 gram
- Monounsaturated Fat: 1.048 grams
- Polyunsaturated Fat: 0.467 gram
- Total Fat: 4.182 grams
- Percentage of Calories From Fat: 12%

Whether you have it for breakfast or dessert, this unbelievably crusty treat is more than satisfying.

6	medium juicy, sweet apples, peeled, cored and thinly sliced
2	cups evaporated skim milk
3/4	cup low-fat ricotta cheese or low-fat creamed cottage cheese
3	large eggs
6	tbsp. sugar
2	tsp. vanilla
	Cinnamon
1	cup instant nonfat dry milk

1. Arrange the apple slices in a 9-inch pie plate, overlapping them in a circular fashion. Bake, uncovered, at 350° for about 25 minutes, or until the apples are slightly soft.
2. In a blender jar combine 1 cup of the evaporated milk and the cheese, eggs, sugar and vanilla and whirl until smooth. Stir in the remaining 1 cup evaporated milk and 1/4 teaspoon of the cinnamon by hand.
3. Pour this mixture over the apples very slowly, not disturbing their arrangement. Sprinkle the dry milk evenly across the top and dust with more of the cinnamon.
4. Bake, uncovered, for about 30 minutes, or until browned, covering if necessary. The center should be custardlike and firm when pressed.
5. Serve warm, at room temperature or even chilled. Let set for a few minutes before cutting.

CHERRY PIE

Nutrition Facts
Number of Servings: 2
Per Serving
- Calories: 308
- Saturated Fat: 2.974 grams
- Monounsaturated Fat: 1.537 grams
- Polyunsaturated Fat: 0.209 gram
- Total Fat: 8.052 grams
- Percentage of Calories From Fat: 24%

A luscious, low-fat version of a popular dessert.

Filling:
1/2 cup evaporated milk (not skim)
1 envelope unflavored gelatin
2 tbsp. sugar
1 tsp. grated fresh lemon rind
2/3 cup low-fat ricotta cheese or low-fat creamed
cottage cheese
1/4 cup yogurt or buttermilk
1–2 tbsp. lime juice
Tiny pinch of salt

Topping:
1/2 envelope unflavored gelatin
3/4 cup diet cherry-flavored soda
1/2 tsp. cherry flavoring (if desired)
1 tbsp. sugar
1/2 cup frozen cherries, thawed and pitted

1. To make the pie filling: Pour the milk into a medium mixing bowl and set it in the freezer for about 1 hour, until crystals begin to form.
2. Pour 1/2 cup water into a saucepan. Add the gelatin to soften. Cook over low heat, stirring constantly, until the gelatin is dissolved. Remove.
3. Add the sugar and the lemon rind. Cool to room temperature.
4. In a bowl combine the cheese, yogurt or buttermilk, lime juice and salt and beat with a rotary mixer until smooth. Clean the beaters and place them in the freezer with the milk.
5. Blend the cheese mixture with the gelatin mixture using a wooden spoon. Chill, stirring occasionally, until it mounds. Do not let it gel. The mixture will look slightly thickened.
6. When the milk in the freezer has formed crystals, beat it with the frozen beaters until stiff, like whipped cream. Beat in the cheese mixture just enough to blend. Pour into a 6- to-8-inch pie plate and chill.
7. To make the cherry topping: Soften the gelatin in the soda. Cook over low heat, stirring, just until the gelatin is dissolved.
8. Remove and blend in the flavoring if using and the sugar. Cool. Drain the cherries and fold in lightly.
9. Chill the topping only until the mixture mounds slightly. Spread over the pie and chill until all is firm.

CLAFOUTI AUX PÊCHES

Nutrition Facts
  Number of Servings: 6
  Per Serving
  • Calories: 361
  • Saturated Fat: 2.07 grams
  • Monounsaturated Fat: 5.548 grams
  • Polyunsaturated Fat: 4.418 grams
  • Total Fat: 12.94 grams
  • Percentage of Calories From Fat: 32%

This clafouti can be prepared with ripe and juicy apricots, bananas or even blueberries.

6   medium ripe peaches, peeled and sliced
7   slices white bread, crusts removed and torn into pieces
2   cups evaporated skim milk
3   large eggs plus 2 additional egg whites (for added moistness)
    Ground nutmeg or mace
6   tbsp. sugar
¼   cup sunflower oil
    Peach flavoring (if desired)
    Almond extract

1. Arrange the peaches in a 9-inch pie plate, overlapping the slices in a circular fashion.
2. Heat the oven to 350°.
3. In a blender jar combine the bread, milk, whole eggs, egg whites, a pinch of the nutmeg or mace, sugar and oil and whirl until smooth. Add the flavoring if using and the extract, ¼ teaspoon at a time to taste.
4. Carefully pour the batter over the peaches to avoid disturbing the arrangement. Bake for about 30 minutes, or until the custard is firm in the center when pressed. Cover with aluminum foil if not done and the top browns too rapidly.
5. Remove and cool. Serve lukewarm or chilled. Sprinkle delicately with more of the nutmeg just before serving.

CRÈME MOCHA (COFFEE CUSTARD)

Nutrition Facts
  Number of Servings: 3
  Per Serving
  • Calories: 184
  • Saturated Fat: 1.191 grams
  • Monounsaturated Fat: 1.354 grams
  • Polyunsaturated Fat: 0.465 gram
  • Total Fat: 3.602 grams
  • Percentage of Calories From Fat: 18%

Whoever said that custard is difficult to make? It takes minutes to whip this up. And if you can find an essence of chocolate and coffee combined, or mocha essence, you will have an even more authentic flavor.

 2   eggs
1 1/2   cups evaporated skim milk
 2   tbsp. sugar or honey
 2   tsp. instant coffee
     Mocha flavoring (if desired)

1. In a blender jar combine the eggs, milk, sugar or honey, and coffee. Whirl at low speed. Add the mocha flavoring if using, starting with about 1/2 teaspoon or more, to taste.
2. Pour the mixture into 3 custard cups. Add 1 inch very hot water to a baking pan and arrange the custard cups in it.
3. Bake at 350° for about 25 to 30 minutes, or until the center is no longer liquid when pressed. Cover with aluminum foil if the custard is browning too rapidly.
4. Immediately remove from the pan and let cool. Eat at room temperature or chilled.

*Savory
Sweets
and
Desserts*
❖

ZABAGLIONE MOUSSE

Nutrition Facts
Number of Servings: 2
Per Serving
- Calories: 124
- Saturated Fat: 0.775 gram
- Monounsaturated Fat: 0.955 gram
- Polyunsaturated Fat: 0.341 gram
- Total Fat: 2.505 grams
- Percentage of Calories From Fat: 18%

Light as a feather, foamy as champagne. All you have to do is get two ordinary pans arranged before you beat the eggs. This pan method is called *bain-marie.*

2   large eggs, separated
4   tbsp. sugar
1   cup diet cream soda, at room temperature
2   tsp. rum flavoring

1. If necessary, improvise a double boiler by arranging a top pan to sit in a bottom pan of simmering water. A 10-inch skillet will do for the bottom pan. Use about 2 cups water. Set another, smaller skillet or a wide, shallow saucepan in the water.
2. When ready to serve this dessert, beat the egg whites in a mixing bowl until stiff. In another bowl beat the egg yolks with the sugar until they are pale yellow.
3. Remove the smaller pan from the water and pour the egg yolks, soda and flavoring into this pan. Heat the water in the bottom pan until it simmers and keep it at the simmering stage.
4. Now put the pan containing the yolk-soda mixture in the water and beat this mixture at high speed until frothy and somewhat firm, like a mousse. This will take about 10 minutes or more, depending on the immersion, heat and other factors.
5. Remove from the heat and immediately fold in the egg whites. Quickly pour into 2 parfait glasses or goblets and eat warm.

CHEESECAKE WITH GRAPES

Nutrition Facts

Number of Servings: 6

Per Serving

- Calories: 233
- Saturated Fat: 1.162 grams
- Monounsaturated Fat: 1.343 grams
- Polyunsaturated Fat: 0.571 gram
- Total Fat: 5.503 grams
- Percentage of Calories From Fat: 22%

In Italy this cheesecake is called torta di ricotta. It is filled with crushed grapes and evokes thoughts of the wine season. And spring.

4	large eggs, separated
1 1/3	cups low-fat ricotta cheese or low-fat creamed cottage cheese
1	cup instant nonfat dry milk
6	tbsp. sugar
	Freshly grated rinds of 1 lemon and 1 orange
1	cup finely chopped seedless green grapes
1/2	cup yogurt or buttermilk
1	tbsp. vanilla
3	cups whole grapes for garnish

1. In a mixing bowl beat the egg whites with a rotary beater until very stiff peaks form.
2. In a different bowl combine the egg yolks, cheese, dry milk, sugar, lemon and orange rinds and chopped grapes and whip with the beater until smooth. Blend in the yogurt or buttermilk and vanilla. Gently fold the egg whites evenly into this mixture.
3. Coat a 9-inch nonstick cake pan with canola oil spray. Pour the mixture into this pan and bake at 400° for about 20 to 25 minutes, or until the center is firm. To prevent drying, do not overbake.
4. Turn onto a serving platter and surround with the whole grapes. Eat at room temperature or chilled.

Savory Sweets and Desserts

❖

157

STRAWBERRY SKILLET SOUFFLÉ

Nutrition Facts
Number of Servings: 2
Per Serving
- Calories: 220
- Saturated Fat: 2.865 grams
- Monounsaturated Fat: 2.628 grams
- Polyunsaturated Fat: 1.135 grams
- Total Fat: 7.677 grams
- Percentage of Calories From Fat: 32%

This puffy omelette has the virtues of a soufflé but takes only minutes to make and serve. And eat!

1	cup sliced strawberries
1/8	tsp. almond flavoring
2	tbsp. sugar
2	large eggs, separated
2	tsp. arrowroot or cornstarch
1/3	cup instant nonfat dry milk
1–2	tsp. rum flavoring
1	tsp. butter

1. In a mixing bowl combine the strawberries, almond flavoring and 1 tablespoon of the sugar. Mix lightly and reserve.
2. Lightly coat the bottom of a 10-inch nonstick skillet with canola oil spray.
3. In a bowl beat the egg whites until they form very stiff, moist peaks, gradually adding the arrowroot or cornstarch as you quickly beat in the dry milk, the remaining 1 tablespoon sugar, rum flavoring and egg yolks.
4. Put the skillet over a low burner and, when warm, pour the egg mixture evenly into the pan. Cover for 2 minutes. Check for doneness: The mixture should be cooked on the outside but slightly *baveuse*, or moist, on the inside.
5. Arrange the strawberries along the center, fold over and slide onto a serving plate. Spread with the butter. Eat at once.

APPLE-OATMEAL MUFFINS

Nutrition Facts
  Number of Servings: 3
  Per Serving
  • Calories: 172
  • Saturated Fat: 0.756 gram
  • Monounsaturated Fat: 0.949 gram
  • Polyunsaturated Fat: 0.676 gram
  • Total Fat: 2.84 grams
  • Percentage of Calories From Fat: 15%

An American tradition, these muffins are puffy and warm and filled with fiber!

1	large egg
1	tbsp. buttermilk
1	tsp. vanilla
3	tbsp. uncooked oats
1/3	cup instant nonfat dry milk
3	tbsp. sugar
1/4	tsp. baking soda
	Pinch of cream of tartar
	Cinnamon
1	medium unpeeled apple, cored and minced

1. Preheat the oven to 400°.
2. In a blender jar combine the egg, buttermilk, vanilla, oats, dry milk, 1 1/2 tablespoons of the sugar, baking soda and cream of tartar. Whirl until smooth. Add the remaining 1 1/2 tablespoons sugar and the cinnamon to taste.
3. Fold the minced apples into the batter evenly.
4. Lightly coat muffin cups or individual custard cups with canola oil spray. Spoon the mixture into 3 large cups or 6 smaller cups.
5. Bake for 12 to 15 minutes, or until puffed and golden brown. To prevent drying, do not overbake. Eat warm or chilled.

Savory
Sweets
and
Desserts
❖
159

BLUEBERRY-BRAN MUFFINS

Nutrition Facts
Number of Servings: 3
Per Serving
- Calories: 167
- Saturated Fat: 3.05 grams
- Monounsaturated Fat: 1.87 grams
- Polyunsaturated Fat: 0.698 gram
- Total Fat: 6.133 grams
- Percentage of Calories From Fat: 29%

Warm and fruity and full of fiber, these muffins can also be a perfect breakfast for a cold winter Sunday morning.

1	large egg
1	tbsp. yogurt
1	tsp. vanilla
3	tbsp. bran cereal
1/3	cup instant nonfat dry milk
3	tbsp. sugar, fructose or honey
1/4	tsp. baking soda
	Pinch of cream of tartar
	Cinnamon
1/2	cup small fresh or frozen blueberries or minced cherries, drained
1	tbsp. butter

1. Preheat the oven to 400°.
2. In a blender jar combine the egg, yogurt, vanilla, cereal, dry milk, 1 tablespoon of the sugar, fructose or honey, baking soda and cream of tartar. Whirl until smooth. Add the remaining 2 tablespoons sugar, fructose or honey and the cinnamon to taste.
3. With a spatula or spoon fold the blueberries or cherries evenly into the batter. Spoon this mixture into nonstick muffin cups or individual custard cups to make either 3 large or 6 small muffins.
4. Bake for 12 to 15 minutes, or until golden brown and puffy. To prevent drying, do not overbake. Spread with the butter and eat warm.

BANANA BREAKFAST SOUFFLÉ

Nutrition Facts
Number of Servings: 4
Per Serving
- Calories: 330
- Saturated Fat: 4.297 grams
- Monounsaturated Fat: 3.16 grams
- Polyunsaturated Fat: 1.05 grams
- Total Fat: 9.769 grams
- Percentage of Calories From Fat: 26%

A very conventional dessert can also be a breakfast delight.

2	tbsp. cornstarch
1	cup evaporated skim milk
	Ground nutmeg
4	tbsp. sugar
4	medium very ripe bananas
4	large eggs, separated
1/4–1/2 tsp.	coconut flavoring (if desired)
1/4–1/2 tsp.	banana flavoring (if desired)
4	tsp. butter

1. In a saucepan dissolve the cornstarch in the milk with a pinch of the nutmeg. Cook over medium heat, stirring constantly, until thickened. Remove from the heat, stir in the sugar and pour into a bowl.
2. Slice the bananas into a blender jar and add the egg yolks. Whirl until smooth.
3. Combine the banana mixture with the cream sauce and stir in the coconut and banana flavorings if using to taste. Reserve.
4. Beat the egg whites in a mixing bowl until they form stiff but moist peaks. Fold into the sauce evenly.
5. Lightly coat a 4- to 6-cup soufflé dish with canola oil spray and spoon the mixture into this dish. Bake at 375° for about 20 to 25 minutes, or until the center is firm. To prevent drying, do not overbake.
6. Spread with the butter and more of the nutmeg, if desired.

*Savory
Sweets
and
Desserts*
❖

BLUEBERRY CREPE

Nutrition Facts
Number of Servings: 1
Per Serving
- Calories: 365
- Saturated Fat: 4.362 grams
- Monounsaturated Fat: 3.722 grams
- Polyunsaturated Fat: 1.689 grams
- Total Fat: 11 grams
- Percentage of Calories From Fat: 27%

One of my daughter's favorites! She claims that this crepe tastes even richer than conventional ones. Truly a lot of food for the ravenous.

¹/₂	cup fresh or frozen blueberries
1	tsp. vanilla
2	tbsp. sugar
1	large egg
¹/₄	cup yogurt
1	slice multigrain bread, torn into pieces
¹/₄	tsp. ground cardamom (if desired but preferable)
1	tsp. butter

1. In a saucepan combine the blueberries, vanilla and 1 tablespoon of the sugar. Cover barely with water and bring to a boil over medium heat. Cook, uncovered and stirring often, until the consistency of preserves. Remove, cover and keep warm.
2. In a blender jar combine the egg, yogurt, bread and the remaining 1 tablespoon sugar. Whirl until smooth. Add the cardamom to taste.
3. Lightly coat a 10-inch nonstick skillet with canola oil spray. Heat the pan over medium-low heat.
4. Pour in the batter, tilting the pan to evenly distribute the mixture. Lift the edge with a spatula and turn the crepe only when it's brown flecked, or it may tear. Cook the other side.
5. Spread the fruit in the center and roll up. Spread the butter over the crepe and eat warm.

BANANA-CORN MUFFINS

Nutrition Facts
Number of Servings: 2
Per Serving
- Calories: 266
- Saturated Fat: 3.413 grams
- Monounsaturated Fat: 2.263 grams
- Polyunsaturated Fat: 0.868 gram
- Total Fat: 7.305 grams
- Percentage of Calories From Fat: 24%

Another muffin good enough for dessert or for an old-fashioned, hearty breakfast.

3	tbsp. yellow cornmeal
1	large egg
1/3	cup instant nonfat dry milk
1/4	tsp. baking soda
	Pinch of cream of tartar
	Ground ginger
1/4	tsp. coconut flavoring or vanilla
2	tbsp. sugar
1	medium ripe banana
2	tsp. butter

1. Preheat the oven to 400°.
2. In a blender jar combine all of the ingredients except the banana and butter, adding the ginger to taste. Whirl until smooth.
3. Mash the banana with a fork or chop it into small chunks. Stir the banana into the batter.
4. Spoon the batter into 6 small nonstick muffin cups or 3 custard cups lightly coated with canola oil spray. Bake for 12 to 15 minutes, or until golden and puffed. To prevent drying, do not overbake.
5. Spread the butter over the muffins and eat warm.

*Savory
Sweets
and
Desserts*
❖
163

WHOLE-WHEAT ZUCCHINI BREAD

Nutrition Facts
Number of Servings: 2
Per Serving
- Calories: 253
- Saturated Fat: 3.473 grams
- Monounsaturated Fat: 2.417 grams
- Polyunsaturated Fat: 1.072 grams
- Total Fat: 8.126 grams
- Percentage of Calories From Fat: 28%

A new tradition: a vegetable as a sweet treat.

1	egg
2	slices whole-wheat bread, torn into pieces
1/4	cup evaporated skim milk
2	tbsp. apple juice
1/3	cup instant nonfat dry milk
	Pinch of ground nutmeg
	Pinch of cinnamon
2	tbsp. brown sugar
1/4	tsp. baking soda
	Pinch of cream of tartar
1	cup grated zucchini
2	tsp. butter

1. Preheat the oven to 400°.
2. In a blender jar combine all of the ingredients except the zucchini and butter and whirl until smooth. With a wooden spoon or spatula combine the zucchini evenly with the egg mixture.
3. Coat a 2-cup nonstick baking dish with canola oil spray. Spoon the batter into this dish and bake for about 12 to 15 minutes, or until golden and puffy. To prevent drying, do not overbake. Remove from the baking dish and dot with the butter.

CARROT-GINGER CORN BREAD

Nutrition Facts
  Number of Servings: 2
  Per Serving
  • Calories: 247
  • Saturated Fat: 3.378 grams
  • Monounsaturated Fat: 2.271 grams
  • Polyunsaturated Fat: 0.851 gram
  • Total Fat: 7.207 grams
  • Percentage of Calories From Fat: 26%

Shredded carrots, spices and sugar in a corn batter are hearty fare. Quick and easy, too.

1	egg
1/4	cup evaporated skim milk
2	tbsp. yogurt
1/3	cup instant nonfat dry milk
1/4	tsp. ground ginger
	Pinch of allspice
2	tbsp. brown sugar
3	tbsp. corn flour or cornmeal
1/4	tsp. baking soda
	Pinch of cream of tartar
1	large carrot, finely shredded
2	tsp. butter

1. Preheat the oven to 400°.
2. In a blender jar combine all of the ingredients except the carrots and butter, starting with the egg and evaporated milk. Whirl until smooth. Remove from the blender and add the carrots, mixing evenly.
3. Lower the oven temperature to 350°.
4. Lightly coat a 2-cup nonstick baking dish with canola oil spray. Spoon the carrot mixture into the baking dish and bake for about 12 to 15 minutes, or until puffed and golden. To avoid dryness, do not overbake.
5. Remove from the oven and spread the butter over the bread. Eat warm.

Savory Sweets and Desserts
❖

RECIPE INDEX

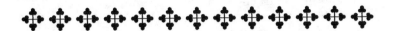

N

O

P

Q

R

S